Medical Management
of the
Home Care Patient

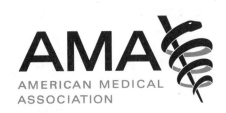

AMA
AMERICAN MEDICAL
ASSOCIATION

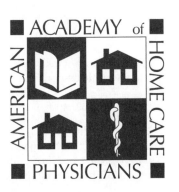

AMERICAN ACADEMY of HOME CARE PHYSICIANS

Additional copies of this book may be ordered by calling 800-621-8335 or from the secure AMA web
site at www.amabookstore.com. Refer to product number OP 221212.

ISBN 978-1-60359-740-1

Citation Statement:
Cornwell T and Schwartzberg JG, eds. *Medical Management of the Home Care Patient:
Guidelines for Physicians*. 4th ed. Chicago, IL: American Medical Association and American
Academy of Home Care Physicians; 2012.

MEDICAL MANAGEMENT OF THE HOME CARE PATIENT: GUIDELINES FOR PHYSICIANS

The information in this monograph is provided to assist physicians in providing care to acute and chronically ill patients in their own homes.

This monograph is not intended as a standard of medical care, nor should it be used as a substitute for physicians' clinical judgment. This material is provided for informational and educational purposes only. None of this monograph's materials should be construed as legal advice nor used to resolve legal problems. If legal advice is required, physicians are urged to consult an attorney who is licensed to practice in their state.

For further information about this monograph, please contact:
Joanne G. Schwartzberg, MD
Director, Aging and Community Health
American Medical Association
515 North State Street
Chicago, IL 60654

Continuing Medical Education Information

Accreditation Statement: The American Medical Association is accredited by the Accreditation Council for Continuing Medical Education to provide continuing medical education for physicians.

Designation Statement: The American Medical Association designates this enduring material for a maximum of *3.5 AMA PRA Category 1 Credits*™. Physicians should claim only the credit commensurate with the extent of their participation in the activity.

Target audience: This activity is designed for all physicians (primary care and specialists) who provide home care visits and/or whose patient population includes patients who would benefit from home care as an option. It is also appropriate for residents in multiple fields.

Statement of competencies: This activity will address the following Accreditation Council for Graduate Medical Education/American Board of Medical Specialties (ACGME/ABMS) competencies: patient care; medical knowledge; interpersonal and communication skills; professionalism; systems-based practice; and interdisciplinary teamwork.

Learning objectives: As a result of participating in this activity, physicians will be able to:

1) Describe the scope of home care and the populations that use it.

2) Describe the physician's role in home care and responsibilities in development and oversight of the home care plan.

3) Determine the appropriateness of a patient for home care.

4) Determine how, when and what services need to be implemented to provide quality care for the patient at home (home health services, homemaker, private duty, durable medical equipment (DME), palliative care and hospice, Veterans Administration services, telehealth, etc.)

5) Explain how quality care transitions and coordinated home care services can reduce hospital admissions.

6) Describe medical ethics and legal and regulatory issues pertaining to the home care patient.

Disclosure:

The content of this activity does not relate to any product of a commercial interest as defined by the ACCME; therefore, neither the planners nor the faculty have relevant financial relationships to disclose.

Instructions for claiming *AMA PRA Category 1 Credits*™

To facilitate the learning process, we encourage the following method for physician participation: Read the material in the *Medical Management of the Home Care Patient: Guidelines for Physicians*, complete the CME Questionnaire and Evaluation, and then fax or mail the questionnaire, evaluation, and CME credit claim form to:

Joanne G. Schwartzberg, MD
Director, Aging and Community Health
American Medical Association
515 North State Street
Chicago, IL 60654
Fax: 312-464-4111

A score of 70 percent or greater is required to pass and receive
AMA PRA Category 1 Credits™.
An AMA Continuing Education Program
Release Date- 3/15/2012
Expiration Date- 3/15/2015

TABLE OF CONTENTS

PREFACE

The American Medical Association (AMA) convened the first Home Care Advisory Panel in 1987 with the goal of increasing the involvement of physicians in home care. That panel produced the first edition of the *Guidelines for the Medical Management of the Home Care Patient*, which was published in 1992 in collaboration with the U.S. Administration on Aging. This fourth edition, *Medical Management of the Home Care Patient: Guidelines for Physicians*, has been made possible by the collaboration between the AMA and the American Academy of Home Care Physicians (AAHCP) and is primarily the work of AAHCP Board Members, assisted by others. We gratefully acknowledge the following:

Thomas Cornwell, MD, Editor
Medical Director and Founder
HomeCare Physicians
Central DuPage Hospital
Winfield, IL

Joanne G. Schwartzberg, MD, Assistant Editor
Director of Aging and Community Health
American Medical Association
Chicago, IL

Alan P. Abrams, MD, MPH
Medical Director
Geriatric Division
The Cambridge Health Alliance
Boston, MA

C. Gresham Bayne, MD
Chairman and Founder
The Call Doctor Medical Group, Inc
San Diego, CA

Peter A. Boling, MD
Professor of Medicine
Virginia Commonwealth University
MCV Campus Director: MCV House Calls,
MCV Long Term Care, and MCV Campus
Geriatrics Section
Richmond, VA

Michael Cantor, MD, JD
Quality Medical Director
New England Quality Care Alliance (NCEQCA)
Assistant Professor of Medicine
Tufts University School of Medicine

Thomas Edes, MD, MS
Director Geriatrics and Extended Care
Office of Clinical Operations
U.S. Department of Veterans Affairs
Washington, DC

Brent T. Feorene, MBA
President
House Call Solutions
Westlake, OH

Ashley Harris, MD
Geriatric Medicine Fellow
Harvard Geriatric Medicine Fellowship Program
Beth Israel Deaconess Medical Center
Boston, MA

Jennifer Hayashi, MD
Director, Elder House Call Program
Johns Hopkins Bayview Medical Center
Johns Hopkins University School of Medicine
Baltimore, MD

Yasmin Issa, MD
Geriatric Medicine Fellow
Harvard Geriatric Medicine Fellowship Program
Beth Israel Deaconess Medical Center
Boston, MA

Kathy Kemle, MS, PA-C, DFAAPA
Assistant Professor
Geriatrics Division
Mercer University School of Medicine
Medical Center of Central Georgia
Macon, GA

James E. Lett II, MD, CMD
National Transitions of Care Coalition (NTOCC)
National Advisory Board

Bruce Leff, MD
Professor of Medicine
Division of Geriatric Medicine
Johns Hopkins University School of Medicine
Baltimore, MD

Russell C. Libby, MD
Virginia Pediatric Group
American Pediatric Consultants
Fairfax, VA

Mel Christopher Magboo, MD
Geriatric Specialty Care
Medical Director
Rosewood Rehabilitation Center
Medical Director
Circle of Life Hospice
Reno, NV

Marjo Magboo, BSN, RN, MBA, WCC
Director of Clinical Nursing
Home Care Plus Home Health Care Agency
Reno, NV

Steven L. Phillips, MD
Geriatric Specialty Care
Reno, NV

Edward Ratner, MD
Associate Professor
Department of Medicine
University of Minnesota Medical School
Minneapolis, MN

Jean A. Yudin, MSN, RN, CS
Director
Schnabel House Call Program
University of Pennsylvania
Philadelphia, PA

The editors and authors gratefully acknowledge the work of:

Kelly Towey, MEd
Consultant
American Medical Association
Chicago, IL

Constance F. Row, LFACHE
Executive Director
American Academy of Home Care Physicians
Edgewood, MD

Jessica E.Quintilian, CHES
Assistant Executive Director
American Academy of Home Care Physicians
Edgewood, MD

We appreciate the assistance of reviewers Alejandro Aparicio, MD, FACP, Paul Chiang, MD, Thomas Lally MD, Steve Landers, MD, Linnea Nagel, MPAS, PA-C, Ancy Zacharia, APN, Susan Levitt BS, RN and Gary Swartz, JD. Thanks to following: Norene Jenkins who updated the Resources chapter, Marsha Meyer for her copy editing and Mark Evans, PhD for his assistance with the continuing medical education component of this book. A special thanks also to Edward Ratner, MD who made extensive edits to the text.

INTRODUCTION

Over the next several decades, the patient's home will become the principal venue for the delivery of an array of health care services, ranging from long-term care to acute hospital-level care and everything in between. This move from hospitals, clinics, and other facilities to the home is being driven by several ever-strengthening secular trends: the rapid aging of the U.S. population, epidemics of chronic disease and multimorbidity, technological advances, health care consumerism, rapidly escalating health care costs[1] and recent health care reform efforts that culminated in the passage of the federal Patient Protection and Affordable Care Act (PPACA) of 2010, which included the Independence at Home Act (IAH).

This monograph describes the medical management of the home care patient in its myriad aspects. Interestingly, "home care" is a deceptively simple term that belies its clinical complexity and semantic challenges. Home care describes a vast array of services ranging from family members balancing the checkbook of a mildly demented parent, to nurse practitioners making postnatal visits to new parents, to skilled physical therapists providing services to a recently discharged stroke patient, to physicians managing a ventilator-dependent patient in that patient's living room.

All of the home care activities described above incur costs in some way, which are covered by an array of payers (including out-of-pocket payments by patients and their families) and complex, often conflicting coverage policies and regulations. In fact, because home care encompasses such a wide variety of activities, it is commonly described in the context of multiple frameworks, with substantial overlap across frameworks. It is critical for the readers of this text to be familiar with the types of home care and their associated terminology and funding sources in the U.S. health care system. As they say at the ballpark, "you can't tell the players without a scorecard." This introductory chapter briefly describes types of home care organized by (1) care provider, (2) care acuity, and (3) payer of care. The Table provides an overview of these frameworks.

TYPES OF HOME CARE BY PROVIDER

At its most fundamental level, home care is assistance provided to a person at home by a family member or friend. This *informal caregiving* may be as simple as running an occasional errand for an older adult who no longer drives a car, or as intensive as 24-hour supervision and hands-on personal care for a younger adult with severe developmental disability. Area agencies on aging can be an excellent resource for patients and families to learn about available support services and resources in their community. When the same services are provided by individuals who receive payment for them, they are considered *formal caregiving*. This type of caregiving may be provided by family members, neighbors, friends or agency direct care workers, all paid by community or state programs. It may also be provided by professionals through a home care agency. Skilled home care generally describes services provided by health care professionals who have completed higher-level formal training and licensing in a particular health care discipline. Skilled care is commonly provided by nurses, rehabilitation therapists (physical, occupational, or speech therapy), and social workers in the context of Medicare-certified home health agencies (HHA). Medicare regulation requires the primary physician to certify that the patient's clinical condition supports his or her homebound status and need for skilled services on an intermittent (not continuous) basis. At the same time, hands-on personal care, which is not considered skilled care but can have significant impact on a patient's quality of life and function, can be provided by HHA aides while the patient is receiving skilled services.

Medical house calls are another important mode of health care delivery to patients who are temporarily or permanently homebound. Physicians and advanced practice clinicians (nurse practitioners and physician assistants) working with physicians can provide at home many of the same routine and urgent medical services available in a typical office practice, thus avoiding unnecessarily burdensome office or emergency department visits, or even hospitalizations and readmissions. When hospitalization is appropriate, some health systems now provide high-level acute care through *hospital-at-home* programs that result in equivalent or superior outcomes at lower costs when compared to usual in-hospital care for appropriate patients with selected diagnoses.[2] Finally, *home hospice* incorporates palliative medical, social, and spiritual care by an interdisciplinary clinical team that works with the patient and informal caregivers to prevent suffering, relieve symptoms, and promote a peaceful and dignified death at home.

TYPES OF HOME CARE BY ACUITY

An alternative framework to describe home care is by the intensity or level of care provided. *Acute care* is by definition the purview of hospital-at-home programs that commonly manage patients with hemodynamically stable congestive heart failure exacerbation, community-acquired pneumonia, and other conditions at home. Moreover, some acute or urgent care may be provided by house call programs or HHAs when it is safe and consistent with the patient's goals. For example, an elderly patient with delirium from an acute urinary tract infection resulting in a noninjurious fall may be reasonably managed at home with oral antibiotics and nursing visits over several days to assess clinical stability and provide caregiver education, all under the supervision of a physician. In this scenario, as well as inpatient or hospital-at-home settings, *post-acute skilled home care* remains an important part of the continuum of care and recovery in the current era of high hospital volumes and rapid turnover of inpatient beds. Indeed, a small but growing number of medical centers are now developing *transitional care* programs that include telephone contact and home visits from advance practice clinicians, nurses, social workers and other skilled personnel to bridge the often-dangerous gap between the inpatient hospital and outpatient medical follow-up. Outpatient medical follow-up can then be provided for appropriate patients through medical house calls, and other components of day-to-day longitudinal care (sometimes called *community-based care*) may be provided by an assortment of different sources depending on insurance and other resources. Specifically, Medicare-certified HHAs may provide ongoing skilled care for patients with chronic conditions such as indwelling urinary catheters or pernicious anemia requiring vitamin B12 injections. Private-duty agencies provide personal care and homemaking services for patients who are able and willing to pay for them privately, or "out-of-pocket", or are eligible to receive such services through Medicaid or other state programs.

TYPES OF HOME CARE BY PAYER

A common theme underlying the frameworks of home care described above is that payment, in many instances, drives care provision. Medicare is the dominant payer for skilled home health services and commercial payers often follow Medicare's lead in payment issues. Medicare Part A or B covers skilled home care provided by Medicare-certified HHAs for patients who have Medicare and meet specific criteria for being "homebound." Medicare does not pay for long-term personal or "custodial" care needed by patients who are dependent in the basic activities of daily living. This type of care is covered during each episode of skilled care, but only during the time that the skilled care is needed. Ongoing custodial care at home may be covered by Medicaid in some states, but requires patients to exhaust their personal financial resources to become eligible or to meet specific Medicaid disability criteria. Personal financial resources can be used to pay directly for formal caregiving or for long-term care insurance that may cover some or all of the costs of in-home services. The Figure shows on the next page the percentage of home care costs covered by each of these major payers, as well as the small percentage covered by various local programs and the Veterans Administration.[3]

SUMMARY

"Home care" denotes a wide variety of activities that all have in common the goal of providing medical or functional support to patients in their own homes. This fourth edition of *Medical Management of the Home Care Patient* is designed to help clinicians traverse the above described home health landscape. It describes in detail the various elements of home health care that the practicing clinician needs to understand and manage effectively in order to provide high quality, patient-centered care at home. Every chapter has been updated, and new chapters discuss transitions in care and their importance in reducing readmissions and the Veterans Administration's Home Based Primary Care Program.

FIGURE National Health Care Home Care Expenditures 2009

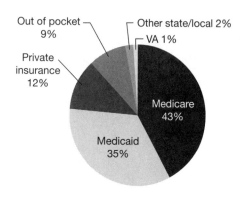

TABLE Types of Home Care

Provider	Time Frame/Acuity	Payer
➤ Informal care-giver	Longitudinal	None
➤ Paid aide	Longitudinal	Medicaid
		Medicare, with concurrent skilled need
		Commercial long-term care insurance
		Private pay
		Veterans Administration

➤ Skilled care/ hospice	Short-term Acute	Medicare Commercial insurance Veterans Administration
➤ Physician/ advance practice clinicians (APC)	Longitudinal Acute	Medicare Medicaid Commercial insurance Private pay Veterans Administration
➤ Hospital-at-home	Acute	Managed care Veterans Administration Demonstration projects Commercial payers

REFERENCES

1. Landers SH. Why health care is going home. *N Engl J Med.* 2010; 363: 1690–1691.

2. Shepperd S, Doll H, Angus RM, Clarke MJ, Iliffe S, Kalra L, Ricauda NA, Tibaldi V, Wilson AD. Avoiding hospital admission through provision of hospital care at home: a systematic review and meta-analysis of individual patient data. *CMAJ.* 2009;180(2):175–182.

3. Centers for Medicare & Medicaid Services web site. http://www.cms.gov/ NationalHealthExpendData, Accessed 2/26/11.

CHAPTER | ONE

Home Care: The First Option

After reading this chapter you should be able to:

1. Describe the scope of home care and the populations that use it

2. Discuss why home care should be the first option for many patients

Fueled by new technologies and shaped by intensifying financial stresses, health care is evolving dramatically. Never have we had more options, and never has health care been more portable. In home care, new diagnostic and therapeutic tools enable us to render comprehensive care, even at the level of intensity found in acute care hospitals. And when care can be safely rendered at home, it is the preferred setting for most people, whether the focus is self-management and preventive maintenance, life-prolonging treatment, short-term recuperation, acute care, chronic long-term care, or palliative care at life's end. Additionally, as has been demonstrated empirically,[1] health care professionals who visit patients at home gain a more accurate, more holistic understanding of patients' needs and capabilities than can be achieved in an office, emergency department or hospital setting. Hospitals, nursing homes, and rehabilitation units all play important roles for people with serious illness but now more than ever, home care is and should be the "first option." This is a vital health policy issue.

Concurrently, demography and epidemiology are driving the growth of home care. As the cohort of baby boomers born shortly after World War II age, the numbers of elderly living with advanced chronic illnesses are forcing rethinking of our health care system. Conditions like cancer and major organ failure, which were once rapidly fatal, now span years. Patients with serious acute illness are discharged from hospitals after a few days or are managed entirely at home. Longitudinal, coordinated care of chronically ill people and concepts like "medical homes" dominate policy discussions.

Yet, despite enhanced technical capabilities and demand for home care, the field has never faced more pressure to demonstrate its value and to evolve so that it can achieve its optimal role in health care. Costs are rising exponentially and striking variances between providers and localities suggest that opportunities exist to improve care while saving money. Home care needs attention and advocacy to attain its deserved place in the larger health care system.

WHAT IS HOME CARE AND WHO USES IT?

Home care is "provision of equipment and services to the patient in the home for the purpose of restoring and maintaining the maximal level of comfort, function, and health."[2] (See Table 1 for goals of home care.) As shown in 2003[3] and 2009[4,5] the agenda of home care encompasses a broad range of services and users (Figures 1 and 2).

Most Medicare-reimbursed home health service use is by groups E and F (Figure 1). Groups C, D and E use more long-term, supportive services funded by Medicaid, long-term care insurance and personal out-of-pocket payments. Groups A and B are more mobile but prefer the convenience of at-home care for prevention (diet, exercise), home diagnostics (pregnancy tests, blood glucose), home monitoring (blood pressure) or cosmetics (teeth whitening).

TABLE 1 The goals of home care

> ➤ Improve health and quality of life through comprehensive primary medical care, nursing, and rehabilitative services

> ➤ Improve recuperation from acute, function-limiting illnesses

> ➤ Promote safe early discharge from institutional care settings

> ➤ Reduce need for hospitalization and nursing home or other institutional placement

> ➤ Provide support for informal caregivers

> ➤ Allow terminally ill patients to die at home in comfort if that is their wish

> ➤ Enhance optimal growth and development of infants and children

> ➤ Enhance the functional potential of patients who depend on supportive devices

> ➤ Foster the maximum possible sustained independence in the setting most patients prefer

FIGURE 1 Home care user categories[5]

		General Population
A No illness (acute or chronic); seek self-help resources		Home Care User Categories
	B	➢ Ambulatory, independent, not "sick" ➢ Some chronic health conditions exist
	C	➢ Younger; function Activities of Daily Living (ADLs) limited by one condition ➢ Not "sick" often, but need continuous ADL support
	D	➢ Older with chronic cognitive or functional impairment ➢ Acutely ill infrequently (low cost), need ADL support
	E	➢ Post-acute care at the end of an illness episode ➢ Return rapidly to a stable condition, home care ends
	F	➢ High co-morbidity & illness burden, "sick", high cost
	Acute care at home	Post-acute, in-home transitional care	Chronic in-home care	End of life care

FIGURE 2 Home care services

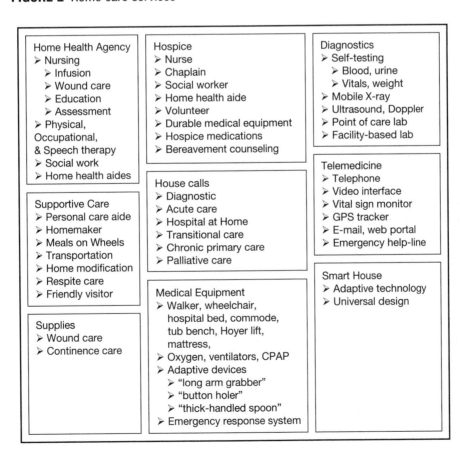

Home Health Agency
➢ Nursing
  ➢ Infusion
  ➢ Wound care
  ➢ Education
  ➢ Assessment
➢ Physical, Occupational, & Speech therapy
➢ Social work
➢ Home health aides

Supportive Care
➢ Personal care aide
➢ Homemaker
➢ Meals on Wheels
➢ Transportation
➢ Home modification
➢ Respite care
➢ Friendly visitor

Supplies
➢ Wound care
➢ Continence care

Hospice
➢ Nurse
➢ Chaplain
➢ Social worker
➢ Home health aide
➢ Volunteer
➢ Durable medical equipment
➢ Hospice medications
➢ Bereavement counseling

House calls
➢ Diagnostic
➢ Acute care
➢ Hospital at Home
➢ Transitional care
➢ Chronic primary care
➢ Palliative care

Medical Equipment
➢ Walker, wheelchair, hospital bed, commode, tub bench, Hoyer lift, mattress,
➢ Oxygen, ventilators, CPAP
➢ Adaptive devices
  ➢ "long arm grabber"
  ➢ "button holer"
  ➢ "thick-handled spoon"
➢ Emergency response system

Diagnostics
➢ Self-testing
  ➢ Blood, urine
  ➢ Vitals, weight
➢ Mobile X-ray
➢ Ultrasound, Doppler
➢ Point of care lab
➢ Facility-based lab

Telemedicine
➢ Telephone
➢ Video interface
➢ Vital sign monitor
➢ GPS tracker
➢ E-mail, web portal
➢ Emergency help-line

Smart House
➢ Adaptive technology
➢ Universal design

Home care is appropriate for all consenting patients whose care needs can be safely managed at home when the required time, financial, physical, and emotional resources are considered. Home care benefits millions of people each year. In 2010 the National Association for Home Care reported that about 12 million people used home care in 2009 through about 33,000 provider organizations.[6] Patient need for home care services spans all ages, although it is skewed toward older adults.

The National Home and Hospice Care Survey (NHHCS) has been conducted periodically since 1992 by the Centers for Disease Control and Prevention's National Center for Health Statistics through interviews with home health and hospice agencies. The most recent report[7] indicates that in 2007 there were 1.46 million home health patients on any given day. Table 2 lists the most common home health patient characteristics, while Table 3 gives the most prevalent medical conditions as indicated by surveys of home health patients.

Also important is the degree of disability. Among home health patients, 84% have limitations in at least one Activity of Daily Living (ADLs: bathing, dressing,

TABLE 2 Home health patient characteristics

➤ 69% ≥ 65 years old

➤ 69% lived with family

➤ 64% female

➤ 5% < 18 years old

➤ 8.1% between 18 and 45 years old

➤ 18.6% between 45 and 64 years old

TABLE 3 Most prevalent home health patient diagnoses

➤ Hypertension 41%

➤ Heart disease 31%

➤ Diabetes 31%

➤ Chronic obstructive pulmonary disease 13%

➤ Arthritis 10%

➤ Cancer 9%

➤ Dementia 7%

➤ Stroke 7%

transferring, toileting and eating), 51% had dependencies in four or five ADLs. This reflects a high degree of functional dependency that in turn translates to service needs.

There is an extensive role for physicians in all the different aspects of home care (see also Chapter 2). For most physicians, the first home care services that come to mind are intermittent, short-term skilled nursing or rehabilitation after an acute illness, or medical equipment like wheelchairs, walkers, hospital beds, and oxygen. These services are delivered by tens of thousands of certified organizations ranging from small local businesses to billion dollar national companies and are primarily supported by Medicare and employer-based insurance.

HOME HEALTH SERVICES COVERED UNDER MEDICARE

Medicare-reimbursed skilled home health care has changed dramatically since 1998 (Figure 3). In response to exponential growth (1988-1997), an Interim Payment System was imposed by the 1997 Balanced Budget Act, followed by a Prospective Payment System in 2000. This shifted risk to providers. Services and costs immediately dropped by half[8] then slowly rebounded. The number of users as a percent of Medicare beneficiaries remains lower than in 1997 and visits per episode remain low.

FIGURE 3 Medicare skilled home health care (1996 to 2008)

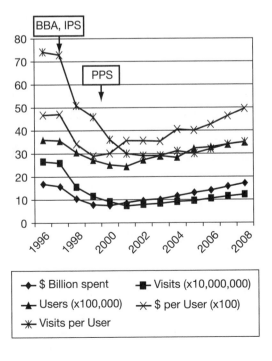

Payment and regulatory reform has produced a change in services since 1997, as shown in Table 4 and in Figure 4. Medicare Part A episodes are shorter, focused on defined, short-term goals, with an increase in therapy visits and a dramatic drop in home health aide services. Social work activity has remained chronically low.

Formal home care is a major industry. In 2008 there were more than one million workers in the field, with 958,000 counted before considering hospital-based and public agencies. Medicare-certified home health agencies employed 290,439 full-time equivalents (FTEs) as home care workers. Of the total 958,000, about 132,000 were registered nurses, 62,000 licensed practical nurses, 24,000 physical therapy staff, 324,000 aides, 7,000 occupational therapists, 16,000 social workers, and almost 400,000 "others."[6] This accounting does not include the personnel involved in the large durable medical equipment domain.

In 2009 the Medicare expenses of around $500 billion constituted about 23% of the more than $2 trillion spent on health care according to MEDPAC (Medicare Payment Advisory Commission).[9] Of Medicare spending, 4% was on home health care, compared with 2% each for hospice and durable medical equipment, 5% for short term nursing home care, 12% for prescription drugs, 12% for physician services, 22% for managed care, 27% for hospital care and 13% for other fee-for-service settings (hospital outpatient, etc.). Costs have been shifting, with drug costs rising rapidly and hospital costs lessening as a percent of the whole (dropping from 39% in 2000 to 27% in 2010). Historically, home health services approached 9% of Medicare spending before the 1997 Balanced Budget Act changes in financing, but has subsequently remained at around 4% for a decade.

About two thirds of new Medicare-reimbursed home health episodes follow hospital inpatient care and on average about 9% of Medicare beneficiaries use home health services each year.[10] Considerable regional variation in service volume exists and concern has been raised about possible inappropriate use in communities where as many as 35% of Medicare beneficiaries receive skilled home health services per year. In 2011 MEDPAC recommended further reductions in Part A home health services payments, while the industry raised concern about quality and access. There is heated debate about the efficiency of care and the "value proposition."

TABLE 4 Medicare-reimbursed home health visits[10] (Average visits during an episode)

Year	1998	2009
➤ Physical therapy	3.1	4.8
➤ Occupational therapy	0.5	1.0
➤ Speech therapy	0.2	0.2
➤ Skilled nursing	14.1	11.8
➤ Social work	0.3	0.1
➤ Home health aide	13.4	3.5

FIGURE 4 Medicare spending is concentrated in certain services and has shifted over time

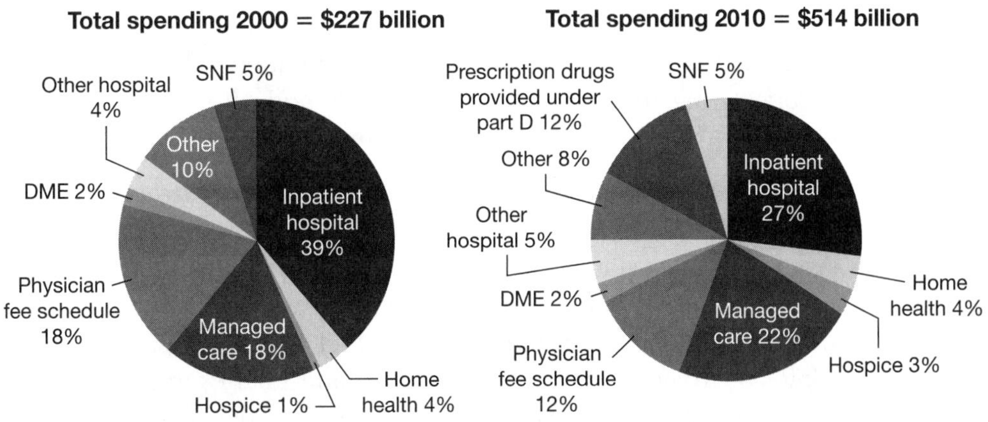

Total spending 2000 = $227 billion   Total spending 2010 = $514 billion

Source: 2012 President's Budget; CMS, Office of the Actuary, 2011.

One third of Medicare Part A home health episodes originate from the community during outpatient care. Home health services are often under-used both at hospital discharge and in the community. For every patient over age 65 in a nursing home, there are three similarly impaired patients in their own homes. An estimated 20% of patients over age 65 have functional impairments with related home care needs that may be unrecognized during a typical office visit.[11] About 15% to 20% of older people living in the community need help for safe ambulation; 7% have three or more deficits in ADLs; and 2% or 3% are essentially bedfast, requiring human help to get out of bed or unable to get out of bed at any time. Too often, they lack longitudinal comprehensive assessment and reassessment with appropriate adjustment of the care plan over time.[12] Likewise, in the hospital setting, studies have indicated that a third of the patients that might benefit from post-acute home health care are not recognized or referred at discharge.[13] Note that the 2010 health care reform legislation (section 3131d) mandates an evaluation of access to home care for low income beneficiaries and those in medically underserved areas.

NON-MEDICARE-COVERED HOME CARE

Another large and important category of home care is longitudinal supportive daily care provided by workers (aides, attendants, companions) who are in the home for several hours per week up to 24 hours per day. These services are funded by Medicaid, long-term care insurance and/or out-of-pocket payments. Thus, services are available predominantly to the affluent and to the poor. For those of moderate means, such services often require use of lifetime savings or borrowing against home equity. This kind of long-term care support is vitally important to help people remain in their homes, including those whose financial assets are limited. Home and community-based long-term care services have grown nationally from 13% of Medicaid long-term care spending in 1997 to 30% in 2000 and 43% in 2007 with proportionate decreases in nursing home spending, reflecting awareness that in-home care is preferable and often less expensive due to the in-kind contributions of unpaid family members.[14]

Unlike Medicare-reimbursed skilled home health care, supportive care services paid for out-of-pocket and by Medicaid show growth that mirrors population changes. Medicaid waivers and other state-specific models of community-based long-term care as an alternative to nursing home care are steadily increasing as shown in Figure 5. Major workforce needs continue. It is not easy to find reliable, capable workers for this sometimes onerous work; training is limited and salaries are low. Quality of service has suffered as a result. New quality measures (Consumer Assessment of Healthcare Providers and Systems [CAHPS®] Home Health Care Survey or HHCAHPS)[15] and alternative financing models are showing promise.[16] Programs such as "Cash and Counseling"[17] are moving this sector forward. Originally the Cash and Counseling Program began as a pilot Medicaid program in 15 states, now this concept of consumer direction has expanded to some non-Medicaid and veteran's programs and is available in some form in over 47 states.

An important subgroup of health system consumers are dually eligible individuals (or "duals") who are covered by both Medicare and Medicaid. Constituting only 15% and 21% respectively of Medicaid and Medicare enrollees, they consume 39% of Medicaid and 36% of Medicare resources. Of the "duals," 3.4 million are under age 65 and 5.5 million are 65 years and older. Average annual costs are around

FIGURE 5 Medicaid-funded home care services (skilled care, personal care, waiver services)

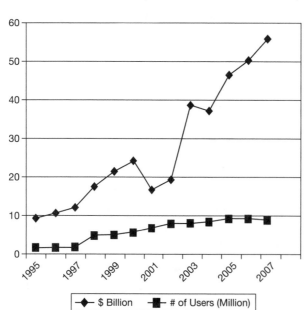

$20,000 per beneficiary.[18] Coordination of care for these often complex patients is now a national priority and a new Federal Coordinated Health Care Office has been created at the Centers for Medicare & Medicaid Services (CMS) to oversee this effort.[19]

HOSPICE

Hospice use has also grown rapidly and is typically provided in the home setting. In 2009 about 70% of those enrolled in hospice were in the home or domiciliary setting.[20] In 2007 slightly more than one million people were discharged from hospice. Noncancer diagnoses are now a slight majority at 57%. There are well over 3,500 operating hospices; the number of users per year has doubled between 2000 and 2009; and at $12 billion in 2009, Medicare hospice care now constitutes about two thirds of Medicare spending on Part A home health care. Average length of stay in hospice has increased from 54 to 86 days but the median duration remains low at 17 days, reflecting reluctance of both patients and providers to choose palliative care.[21] Hospice is now an important part of the final stage of chronic illness care for many U.S. citizens and there is increasingly strong evidence that it facilitates the option of dying at home, which many people prefer.[22]

HOW BROADLY SHOULD HOME CARE BE DEFINED?

To evaluate the cost and value of home care, its boundaries must be defined. The post-acute Medicare benefit and Medicaid long-term care benefits arbitrarily defined a service model and patient population. All such definitions involve both service and user characteristics. Considering the home as the preferred site of health care or "first option," various applications of technology might be considered home care, even when used by healthy ambulatory people with little or no illness burden (Figure 1, Groups A and B). Examples are self-testing for diabetic control, monitoring weight or blood pressure,[23] and exchanging information electronically with health professionals via web portals and e-mail.

Where should the line be drawn? Some technologies are used both by healthy, functional people and by immobile, debilitated individuals and their families. If desired, telemedicine, medication dispensing equipment, robots, and remote data management, even including personal tracking devices like GPS and video monitors, bring the ability to observe and manage every aspect of a person's life at home. "Smart" technology and universal design are adapting future homes to the needs of those with physical or cognitive impairment. Is this home care?

At the far end of the clinical spectrum are items that all analysts would consider components of "home health care": advanced bed surfaces, compact mechanical ventilators, positive-pressure mask ventilation, multi-channel infusion pumps, mobile x-ray and ultrasound equipment, and hand-held point-of-care testing. Such devices make it possible to "medicalize" the home with highly complex care.

Ultimately, by combining self care, long-term supportive care, and the integration of medical house calls into the post-acute and advanced chronic illness care paradigm, "home care" becomes comprehensive, stopping short only of incorporating major surgery, advanced imaging, and intensive care unit treatment. After decades of employing various short-term home care models as a means of post-acute rehabilitation and as a substitute for some portions of hospital-based care, longitudinal, comprehensive primary care at home is being reimagined and incorporated into the health policy dialogue. This is a critical transformation.

It is important to remember that regardless of whether the focus is cure, recovery or chronic maintenance and then palliation in the last months and years of life, effective home-based care requires a collaborative team effort by patient, family, and multiple professionals.

HOW DOES HOME CARE DEMONSTRATE ITS VALUE?

One challenge for home care is "proof of concept." Demonstrating effectiveness in home care is complicated by the diversity of home care programs and the various outcomes measured. Medicare funded the development of a federally mandated outcomes-based measurement and quality improvement method for short-term skilled home health agency care in the late 1990s.[24] Examples of some outcomes are shown in Table 5.

TABLE 5 Examples of measurable home care outcomes

➤ Improvement and/or stabilization in functional status (ADLs)

➤ Improvement and/or stabilization in symptom control, such as dyspnea or pain

➤ Improvement in patient/caregiver management of medications and other treatments

➤ Improvement in patient/caregiver ability to manage equipment

➤ Improvement in knowledge of disease process and signs and symptoms to report

➤ Improvement in knowledge of safety and provision of safe environment

➤ Decrease in utilization of emergency departments and acute/subacute hospitalizations

➤ Decrease in institutional/nursing home placement

A major multi-state national demonstration with about 265,000 intervention patients showed improved risk-adjusted clinical outcomes and impressively reduced hospitalization rates.[25] Specifically, targeted clinical outcomes among 41 available options each improved by 5% to 7% compared with control agency outcomes that were unchanged. Hospitalization was reduced by about 25% over a three-year span. However, the success of these exemplar agencies has not been consistently replicated in nationwide practice during subsequent years. As shown in Figure 3, the past decade has been marked by far fewer visits during an average Part A episode delivered under financial risk. Along with substantial inter-agency variation in system design and a general lack of integration with hospital and medical care providers, these changes are potential causes of the mixed results from the Medicare home health program as a whole. Risk-adjusted acute care hospitalization rates are among 11 publicly reported outcome measures, and are now a focal point of the quality debate.

The June 2011 MEDPAC report[9] reinforces the compelling importance of the costliest health care users, with 14% of Medicare costs supporting 1% of beneficiaries; 25% of costs from the next 4% of users; and 18% from the next 5%. The top 10% together consumed 57% of the budget and the top quarter used 83%. The greatest opportunities and the greatest challenges for home care are in preventing avoidable hospital admissions. Since the 1997 Balanced Budget Act, emergent hospitalization during home care has remained high and relatively constant at 29% of Medicare home health episodes, with many missed opportunities to contain costs and marked inter-agency variation on this performance characteristic. There is a recent hopeful sign: after a sustained national campaign led in part by the Medicare Quality Improvement Organization (QIO) program during the past few years, the national home health care to acute care hospitalization rate had dropped to 26% as reported in July 2011 on http://www.medicare.gov/HomeHealthCompare/search.aspx. However, work remains to be done, and the integration of active physician work on the usual home care team remains an inconsistent but vital element.

Examples from high-performing organizations and innovators clearly show that well-applied, data-driven performance improvement interventions, telemedicine, disease-specific models, and applications of high tech home care such as infusion therapy have substituted for and reduced use of institutional care. Many of these models are discussed in more detail in other chapters of this monograph. The evidence of benefit in home care spans the age spectrum, including studies on children showing safety of early discharge[26] and improved outcomes for children and their mothers[27] that in some cases have shown long-term social benefits.[28] Disease-specific programs have shown benefit for conditions such as chronic lung disease[29] and heart failure.[30] Rigorous randomized, controlled clinical trials have demonstrated that nurse practitioners and physicians working together in short-term transitional care programs following hospitalization[31,32], as well as longitudinal programs such as the Veteran Affairs home-based primary care program,[33] can reduce overall medical care costs in the range of 20% to 50%, if targeted carefully and implemented by experienced teams. "Hospital-at-home" can substitute for institutional care, saving money and enhancing quality[34]; like many successful strategies, efficacy varies among studies.[35]

House calls can also postpone nursing home admission, improve functional outcomes and even reduce the chance of dying.[36,37] New studies are underway such as a program for newly diagnosed childhood diabetes, again emphasizing the value that may be gained from understanding the home setting and the context of illness.[38] This is hard work, and there is not yet a reward system that aligns incentives and encourages growth of these models, although a new concept called Independence at Home is to be tested as part of the 2010 health care reform legislation. (Demonstration web site: http://www.cms.gov/DemoProjectsEvalRpts/MD/itemdetail.asp?filterType=none&filterByDID=-99&sortByDID=3&sortOrder=descending&itemID=CMS1240082&intNumPerPage=10)

SUMMARY

Home care is broad in scope, varied in the focus of its component services and spans the continuum of age, acuity, and intensity from acute and post-acute to chronic care. Advances in technology have expanded the range of home care. At its best, it is the preferred and most cost-effective "first option" for most patients and their families. Continued research and advocacy are needed because unlike hospitals and clinics, home care is unfamiliar to many involved in making policy and determining health care resource allocation, and it is not as well integrated into the overall fabric of health care as it should be. Improved measures of quality and beneficial effect will foster continued growth and dissemination of new and better models of care.

REFERENCES

1. Ramsdell JW, Swart JA, Jackson JE, Renvall M. The yield of a home visit in the assessment of geriatric patients. *J Am Geriatr Soc.* 1989;37:17–24.

2. American Medical Association, Council on Scientific Affairs. Home care in the 1990s. *JAMA.* 1990;263:1241–1244.

3. Levine SA, Boal J, Boling PA. Home care. *JAMA.* 2003;290:1203–1207.

4. Boling PA. The past, present and future of home health care. *Clin Geriatr Med.* 2009; 25(1): xi–xiii.

5. Boling PA. Effects of policy, reimbursement, and regulation on home health care. In: *The Role of Human Factors in Home Health Care: Workshop Summary.* Washington, DC: The National Academies Press; 2010:275–303.

6. National Association for Home Care and Hospice. Basic Statistics about Home Care (Updated 2010). National Association for Home Care and Hospice web site; http://www .nahc.org/facts/. Accessed September 19, 2011.

7. Caffrey C, Sengupta M, Moss A, Harris-Kojetin L, Valverde R. Home health care and discharged hospice care patients: United States, 2000 and 2007. *National Health Statistics Reports; no 38*. Hyattsville, MD: National Center for Health Statistics. 2011.

8. Murkofsky RL, Phillips RS, McCarthy EP, Davis RB, Hamel MB. Length of stay in home care before and after the 1997 Balanced Budget Act. *JAMA*. 2003;289:2841–2848.

9. MEDPAC (Medicare Payment Advisory Commission). *A Data Book. Health Care Spending and the Medicare Program*. Washington DC: Medicare Payment Advisory Commission; 2011. http://www.medpac.gov/documents/Jun11DataBookEntireReport.pdf. Accessed September 19, 2011.

10. MEDPAC (Medicare Payment Advisory Commission). *Report to Congress: Medicare Payment Policy*. Washington, DC: Medicare Payment Advisory Commission; 2011. http:// www.medpac.gov/documents/Mar11_EntireReport.pdf. Accessed September 19, 2011.

11. American Medical Association, Council on Scientific Affairs. American Medical Association white paper on elderly health. *Arch Intern Med*. 1990;150:2459-2472.

12. Boling PA. *The Physician's Role in Home Health Care*. New York, NY: Springer Publishing Co; 1997.

13. Bowles KH, Naylor MD, Foust JB. Patient characteristics at hospital discharge and a comparison of home care referral decisions. *J Am Geriatr Soc*. 2002;50:336–342.

14. Lyons B, Watts MO. *Health Reform Opportunities: Improving Policy for Dual Eligibles. Publication (#7957)*. Kaiser Family Foundation web site. http://www.kff.org. Accessed September 19, 2011.

15. Consumer Assessment of Healthcare Providers and Systems (CAHPS®) Home Health Care Survey web site. https://homehealthcahps.org/. Accessed September 19, 2011.

16. Felix HC, Mays GP, Stewart MK, Cottoms N, Olson M. Medicaid savings resulted when community health workers matched those with needs to home and community care. *Health Aff (Millwood)*. 2011 Jul;30(7):1366–74.

17. Dale S, Brown R, Phillips B, Schore J, Carlson BL. The effects of cash and counseling on personal care services and Medicaid costs in Arkansas. Health Aff (Millwood). 2003 Jul-Dec;Suppl Web Exclusives:W3-566-75.

18. The Henry J. Kaiser Family Foundation. *Kaiser Commission on Medicaid Facts: Dual Eligibles: Medicaid's Role for Low-Income Medicare Beneficiaries, Washington*, DC: The Henry J. Kaiser Family Foundation; May, 2011. www.kff.org. Accessed November 2011.

19. Centers for Medicare and Medicaid Services. *Fact Sheet: People enrolled in Medicare and Medicaid*, May 2011, Centers for Medicare and Medicaid Services web site. http://www.cms .gov. Accessed September 19, 2011.

20. Department of Health & Human Services Office of Inspector General. *Medicare Hospices That Focus On Nursing Faculty Residents*. Department of Health & Human Services Office of Inspector General Web site. http://oig.hhs.gov/oei/reports/oei-02-10-00070.pdf. Accessed July 2011.

21. MEDPAC (Medicare Payment Advisory Commission). *Report to Congress: Medicare payment policy*. Washington, DC: Medicare Payment Advisory Commission; 2011. http://www .medpac.gov/documents/Mar11_EntireReport.pdf. Accessed September 19, 2011.

22. Shepperd S, Wee B, Straus SE. Hospital at home: home-based end of life care. *Cochrane Database Syst Rev* 011 Jul 6;(7):CD009231.

23. Stergiou GS, Bliziotis IA. Home blood pressure monitoring in the diagnosis and treatment of hypertension: a systematic review. *Am J Hypertens.* 2011 Feb;24(2):123–34. Epub 2010 Sep 9.

24. Shaughnessy P, Crisler K, Schlenker R. Measuring and assuring the quality of home health care. *Health Care Financing Rev.* 1994;16:35–65.

25. Shaughnessy PW, Hittle DF, Crisler KS, Powell MC, Richard AA, Kramer AM, et al. Improving patient outcomes of home health care: findings from two demonstrations of outcome-based quality improvement. *J Am Geriatr Soc.* 2002;50:1354–1364.

26. Casiro O, McKenzie ME, McFadyen L, et al. Earlier discharge with community-based intervention for low birth weight infants: a randomized trial. *Pediatrics.* 1993;92;128–133.

27. Kitzman H, Olds DL, Henderson CR Jr, Hanks C, Cole R, Tatelbaum R, McConnochie KM, Sidora K, Luckey DW, Shaver D, Engelhardt K, James D, Barnard K. Effect of prenatal and infancy home visitation by nurses on pregnancy outcomes, childhood injuries, and repeated childbearing. A randomized controlled trial. *JAMA.* 1997 Aug 27;278(8):644–652.

28. Ram FS, Wedzicha JA, Wright J, Greenstone M. Hospital at home for patients with acute exacerbations of chronic obstructive pulmonary disease: systematic review of evidence. *BMJ.* 2004 Aug 7;329(7461):315. Epub 2004 Jul 8.

29. McLean S, Nurmatov U, Liu JL, Pagliari C, Car J, Sheikh A. Telehealthcare for chronic obstructive pulmonary disease. *Cochrane Database Syst Rev.* 2011 Jul 6;(7):CD007718.

30. Rich M, Beckham V, Wittenberg C, et al. A multidisciplinary intervention to prevent the readmission of elderly patients with congestive heart failure. *N Engl J Med.* 1995;333:1190–1195.

31. Naylor MD, Brooten D, Campbell R, Jacobsen BS, Mezey MD, Pauly MV, Schwartz JS. Comprehensive discharge planning and home follow-up of hospitalized elders: a randomized clinical trial. *JAMA.* 1999;281:613–620.

32. Boling PA. Care transitions and home health care. *Clin Geriatr Med.* 2009; 25(1):135–148.

33. Beales JL, Edes T. Veteran's Affairs home based primary care. *Clin Geriatr Med.* 2009 Feb;25(1):149–154, viii–ix.

34. Leff B, Burton L, Mader SL, Naughton B, Burl J, Inouye SK, Greenough WB 3rd, Guido S, Langston C, Frick KD, Steinwachs D, Burton JR. Hospital at home: feasibility and outcomes of a program to provide hospital-level care at home for acutely ill older patients. *Ann Intern Med.* 2005 Dec; 143(11):798–808.

35. Shepperd S, Doll H, Angus RM, Clarke MJ, Iliffe S, Kalra L, Ricauda NA, Tibaldi V, Wilson AD. Avoiding hospital admission through provision of hospital care at home: a systematic review and meta-analysis of individual patient data. *CMAJ.* 2009 Jan 20;180(2):175–182.

36. Stuck AE, Egger M, Hammer A, Minder CE, Beck JC. Home visits to prevent nursing home admission and functional decline in elderly people: systematic review and meta-regression analysis. *JAMA.* 2002 Feb; 287(8):1022–1028.

37. Huss A, Stuck AE, Rubenstein LZ, Egger M, Clough-Gorr KM. Multidimensional preventive home visit programs for community-dwelling older adults: a systematic review and meta-analysis of randomized controlled trials. *J Gerontol A Biol Sci Med Sci.* 2008 Mar; 63(3):298–307.

38. Townson JK, Gregory JW, Cohen D, Channon S, Harman N, Davies JH, Warner J, Trevelyan N, Playle R, Robling M, Hood K, Lowes L. Delivering early care in diabetes evaluation (DECIDE): a protocol for a randomised controlled trial to assess hospital versus home management at diagnosis in childhood diabetes. *BMC Pediatr.* 2011 Jan 19;11:7.

CHAPTER TWO

The Physician's Role in Home Care

After reading this chapter you should be able to:

1. Describe the physician's role in home care and the interdisciplinary team

2. Explain the value of house calls

3. Determine appropriateness of a patient for home care

4. Identify essential assessment areas for evaluating home care patients

Physicians vary in their comfort with referring patients to home care in part because of the vast array of potential services, the multiple organizations that provide pieces of these services, and different federal and state regulatory requirements for physician direction, oversight, and coordination (see Chapter 1, Figure 2). There may be as many different individuals (e.g., health care professionals, direct care workers/aides, administrators, etc.) interacting with the patient at home as in the hospital. However, in the hospital there is an overarching administrative and physical structure that can facilitate communication and coordination, whereas in the home care situation, often the only common elements are the patient/family/caregivers and the physician. The physician's role in the medical management of these complex situations consists of maintaining a well-informed continuous relationship with the patient and overseeing the many different organizations that provide patient services. Also, the physician needs to certify the medical necessity of home services and that federal and state requirements are met. How the physician maintains this "informed continuing relationship" with the homebound patient has not been well defined by tradition or regulation. While for every complex, chronically ill patient in a nursing home there are three similarly impaired patients cared for at home, the actual provision of physician care has been remarkably different in these two settings. The physician's involvement in providing supervision and direct hands-on care for nursing home patients has been determined by Medicare regulation to be at least every 30 days for the first 90 days then every 60 days thereafter. No similar regulatory requirement exists for direct physician care of the patient at home. The difficulty in arranging for these patients to be seen in the office, sometimes requiring a handicap-accessible van or even ambulance transportation, has often led to limited physician hands-on care for these very frail and needy patients.

Increased focus on active physician participation in and accountability for home care and hospice is evident in new federal policy. Under the Affordable Care Act, newly required processes as of January 2011 include mandatory home visits by a hospice physician or nurse practitioner for patients entering the third or subsequent benefit period. Furthermore, as of April 2011 the home health "face to face" visit rule requires that every Medicare Part A new home health episode is certified by a physician who has recently seen the patient (90 days prior to the start of home health care or within 30 days after the start of care) and who documents the medical necessity for home care. Although these policies may sometimes hinder care, they are examples of regulators seeking to increase physician engagement, which has been recognized as a shortcoming for many years.[1] The need for greater physician engagement and team leadership is underscored in many areas of the current health care reform legislation and is specifically required by the Independence at Home Act and the Patient Centered Medical Home models. Health care reform also includes incentives for physicians, practices, HMOs, and other organizations to prevent unnecessary readmissions to the hospital. Because reducing preventable admissions is a national priority, integrating medical services and home health skilled services is critical (see Chapter 8: Care Transitions).[2,3]

IDENTIFYING THE NEED FOR HOME CARE

Home care begins with the physician's recognition that a patient's condition, including his or her medical, psychiatric, functional, and social situation, necessitates care within the home. The physician, in consultation with the patient, family, and other members of the home care team, works to develop and implement a home care treatment plan that may involve a home health agency (HHA), home and community-based services and other resources.[4] The Centers for Medicare & Medicaid Services requires that each patient's individual care plan must be personally reviewed and signed by a physician (allopathic, osteopathic or podiatrist) in order for the HHA services to be covered under the Medicare program.[5] Medicare eligibility criteria are the same whether a referral starts in the office or the hospital: 1) having great difficulty leaving home for anything other than health care and doing so infrequently (homebound); 2) having a skilled care need (for nursing, physical therapy or speech therapy) that can be addressed safely with intermittent care at home—this can be as simple as nursing assessment, teaching and supervision of a care plan for a new or unstable medical condition, or physical therapy after a fall or for a significant new functional deficit; 3) having a physician's order for home health care certifying that the patient's clinical conditions supports the patient's homebound status and need for skilled services; and 4) having a face-to-face visit with the certifying physician. After establishing the medical necessity for home health care, the physician is legally responsible for the supervision and documentation of continuing need for such services.[6]

Prior to initiating home care services, a physician should discuss with the patient his or her role in that patient's care. This includes coordination of care with other physicians, nurse practitioners or physician assistants, the HHA and other community resources, and the services each will provide. Transportation arrangements necessary for continuing monitoring and treatment from the physicians' office and the possibility of providing medical care through house calls should also be discussed. An outline of the physician's role in home care is provided in Table 1.

TABLE 1 The primary physician's role in home care

➤ Identification of the home care needs of the patient (i.e., referring to home health agency when appropriate)

➤ Documentation of Medicare-required face-to-face encounter

➤ Preparing and reassessing the treatment plan

➤ Evaluation of new, acute, or emergent medical problems based on information provided by other team members

➤ Provision for continuity of care in all settings

➤ Communication with the patient, care team members, and physician consultants

➤ Participation in interdisciplinary team and family meetings

➤ Evaluation of quality of care

➤ Documentation in the appropriate medical record

➤ Certification of medical necessity

➤ Making house calls or using health information technology (HIT) such as telehealth and remote patient monitoring when available or appropriate

➤ Provision for 24-hour on-call coverage by a physician

➤ Oversight/evaluation of care transitions

HOUSE CALLS

There are a number of circumstances when a home visit by the physician is appropriate, whether or not home health services are provided. Common reasons that a physician should consider making a house call are outlined in Table 2. Often a house call will serve as the first step in developing a home-based-management plan. While there are important exceptions to this generalization (e.g., pre-operative patient training and evaluation, post-operative follow-up, post-hospital discharge, etc.), house calls can provide information that may be useful or even critical for some acute and most chronic home care situations. Medicare and most other payers will reimburse for services at a rate slightly higher ($10-$30 per visit) than office visits.

Following the initial evaluation, the home care plan may be carried out by the patient alone, but more often it involves family or other caregivers with support from a variety of health care professionals. One current home care model focuses on physician visits with an interdisciplinary approach that involves team meetings to discuss patient progress while reassessing care plans.[7] The physician's direct, physical presence using house calls is often critical in convincing family caregivers that care in the home is possible and acceptable. Often, having a physician available to make a home visit relieves family members' anxiety and prevents unnecessary visits to outpatient clinics and emergency departments. Several changes in the Medicare fee schedule between 1998 and 2006 led to increased payments and more billed physician house calls to patients in private homes and assisted living facilities. The total number of physician house calls increased from 1.6 million (1998) to 4.2 million annually (2010). However,

TABLE 2 Reasons for making a house call

➤ Patient unable to travel to the physician's office due to immobility, cognitive impairment, or psychiatric condition

➤ Request for home visit made by other home health team member, patient, or family member

➤ Need to meet with patient and caregivers to make important decisions

➤ Need for direct observation of patient's environment, patient's functional abilities, or caregiver activities to understand medical issues (e.g., failure of treatments, unexplained symptoms)

➤ Need to meet on-site with community-based providers

➤ Need for direct observation in the home to verify eligibility for third-party reimbursement for services (e.g., homebound status for Medicare Home Health)

➤ Improve care transitions and reduce hospital readmissions

given the number of patients who would benefit from such services, including the estimated 5 million who are homebound, the numbers are still small. The booklet, Making House Calls a Part of Your Practice, published by the American Academy of Home Care Physicians (revised February 2011), is a useful resource for efficiently incorporating house calls into a primary care (or specialty) practice, (www.aahcp.org).

INITIAL EVALUATION FOR HOME CARE

The success of the care plan ultimately depends on the patient or caregiver's ability to carry it out. The physician's support and encouragement are essential factors in patient compliance with the care plan.[8] Appropriate medical management in the home is a function of the physician's skills in optimizing the patient's independence while utilizing medical and social resources to minimize the effects of illness and disability in the patient's daily life. A subtle, but critical distinction between medical management in the home and medical management in the hospital, clinic, or office is the emphasis on the patient's functional abilities, family assistance, and environmental factors. An array of assessments is generally required to evaluate the patient's and/or family caregiver's ability to implement the care plan, including the risk of caregiver burnout. These assessments have proven valuable in both the identification of new medical and psychosocial factors not evident in the office[9,10] and the prevention of further disability.[11,12]

As is the case in any health care setting, the evaluation begins with a comprehensive history and physical examination including functional, cognitive and other assessments, medication review and reconciliation, advance care planning decisions, and appropriate laboratory tests. This process should include a careful assessment of nutritional risk, especially in older patients and patients with chronic illness.[13] The availability of sophisticated testing equipment for in-home use has increased the scope of laboratory tests, but the use of this technology should be tempered by the patient's treatment goals. Beyond the basic medical evaluation, the areas outlined in Table 3 should serve as targets for careful screening during the initial evaluation. The screening assessments should include subjective reports from the patient (and/or family) and the physician's observations during the physical examination. When limitations in daily functioning are identified during the screening process, a more thorough investigation of the underlying process should be completed as described in Table 4. Table 5 lists assistive devices that might be of help for underlying functional impairments. The evaluation process and care plan should also be sensitive to health literacy, as well as cultural and racial issues that can influence outcomes.[14]

TABLE 3 Areas of potential importance for initial home care evaluation

Type of assessment	Specific assessment	Elements to be observed and evaluated
Patient assessments	*Functional assessments* Against the backdrop of the disease process, the physician must assess the patient's ability to perform activities of daily living (ADL) and the more complex instrumental activities of daily living (IADL)	ADL ➤ Ambulating ➤ Toileting ➤ Transferring ➤ Bathing ➤ Feeding ➤ Continence ➤ Dressing IADL ➤ Taking medications appropriately ➤ Handling finances ➤ Using the telephone ➤ Arranging transportation ➤ Preparing meals ➤ Shopping ➤ Doing housework Gait and balance assessment/fall prevention Sensory assessment ➤ Vision ➤ Hearing
	Mental/cognitive assessment Assesses the ability of the patient to follow/ implement the directed care plan	➤ Alcohol or drug use ➤ Cognitive ability and educational development ➤ Recent changes in cognition ➤ Decision-making capacity ➤ Health literacy ➤ Use of medications that affect cognition
	Psychosocial assessment Interventions must be individualized to be effective	➤ Nature and quality of interactions with others ➤ Affect and mood ➤ Cultural, ethnic, or religious influences on health care behavior, beliefs, preferences, and expectations
	Nutritional assessment There is potential for malnutrition in the socially isolated or disabled population	➤ Eating habits: preferences, frequency, and content of meals ➤ Oral health/dental needs ➤ Access to shopping assistance and the ability to purchase and prepare food ➤ Fluid intake ➤ Changes in body weight ➤ Ability to swallow
	Medication use and compliance	➤ All medications (prescription, over-the-counter, herbal and other remedies, and substances of abuse, such as alcohol) present in the home

	A structured approach based on thorough assessment and patient education can reduce adverse drug events	➤ Patient's understanding of the function of medications, desired outcomes, and potential side effects
		➤ History of allergies and adverse drug events
		➤ Written instructions
		➤ Numbers/names of prescribing physicians
		➤ Patient's current regimen and compliance
		➤ Patient's understanding of how to handle medication errors
	Advance care planning	➤ Resuscitation wishes ➤ Health care agents/durable powers of attorney and guardianship
Caregiver assessments	Assessment of burden of caregiving	➤ Caregiving responsibilities (i.e., spouse with Alzheimer's, grandchild, disabled child)
		➤ Number of hours of caregiving work per day
		➤ Nature of tasks to be completed
		➤ Physical and psychological stress related to nature of illness and necessary care
		➤ Caregiver's perception of the need for respite
	Assessment of the caregiver	➤ Acceptance of the responsibility ➤ Willingness and ability to learn and apply knowledge
		➤ Emotional competence, stability ➤ Willingness and ability to implement care plan
		➤ Caregiver's availability ➤ Physical capacity to meet caregiving needs
		➤ History of abusive behaviors ➤ Willingness and ability to work with the care team
		➤ Number of available caregivers ➤ History of family relationships and traditions
Environmental assessment	➤ Safety of the area for patient care activities (barriers, hazards, cleanliness, overcrowding)	
	➤ Access to emergency services; emergency response/alert systems	
	➤ Alternative source of electricity if life-supporting equipment is needed	
	➤ Adaptations needed in terms of special equipment, furniture arrangement, remodeling	

(Continued)

TABLE 3 *Continued*

Type of assessment	Specific assessment	Elements to be observed and evaluated
	➤ Telephone availability and accessibility	➤ Access to toilet, food, water, medication
	➤ Adequate fire safety plan	➤ Adequate storage space for supplies and equipment
	➤ Adequate space for caregivers	➤ Transportation accessibility
	➤ Stability of housing situation	
Community assessment	➤ Safety of neighborhood for patient care	
	➤ Communication as needed with local police, fire, utilities, highway departments, and emergency medical services	
	➤ Community resources—Eldercare services; legal, mental health, social services available at home	
Financial assessment	➤ Eligibility for patient to receive services under Medicare/Medicaid/Veterans Administration or other public programs	
	➤ Resources for private funding for necessary care, including insurance	
	➤ Impact on family resources from inadequate coverage	
	➤ Ability of patient and/or caregivers to manage finances	

TABLE 4 Assessing the level of functional disability

Level of functional disability
➤ Patient is independent
➤ Patient needs minimal assistance
➤ Patient needs moderate assistance
➤ Patient is dependent
Determine the cause of the impairment
➤ Temporary vs. permanent physical limitation
➤ Uncontrolled pathophysiologic process (i.e., congestive heart failure)
➤ Pain
➤ Lack of motivation
➤ Cognitive and psychiatric impairment

Determine the methods to reduce the level of disability

➤ Rehabilitation services

➤ Pharmacotherapy

➤ Psychotherapy

➤ Assistive devices

➤ Increased formal or informal caregiving

➤ Skills training for caregivers

TABLE 5 Assistive devices for functional impairments

➤ Ambulation: Walker (no wheels, two wheels, four wheels), cane, standard wheel chair, scooter, electric wheel chair, stair lifts

➤ Transferring: Lift chair, Hoyer lift, hospital bed with trapeze, transfer board, floor to ceiling grab pole

➤ Eating: Large-handled utensils, rocker knives, cuff that attaches utensil to hand, cups with T-shaped handle or two-sided handles, sippy cups, adhesive place-mats, plate guards

➤ Dressing: Button hook, dressing stick to help put pants on, sock aide, long shoe horn, Velcro fasteners, reacher, zipper puller, elastic shoelaces

➤ Bathing: Bath chair or bench, hydraulic bath chair lift, rubber mat, grab bars, walk in (wheel in) shower, long-handled brushes, inflatable sink for shampooing in bed, urinal

➤ Toileting: Bedside commode, raised toilet seat, grab bars

➤ Medication management devices

THE PHYSICIAN AND THE HOME CARE TEAM

Home care is a team endeavor and physicians have a number of distinct and important roles within the interdisciplinary home health team. These roles can be challenging for physicians who are accustomed to face-to-face contact with interdisciplinary team members in the hospital or office practice setting. Communicating complex information and coordinating care from diverse personnel via telephone, fax or email can be very difficult. Clearly defining the roles and responsibilities of each team member can improve the ability of the physician to participate effectively in the home care process. High-level involvement by a physician in the oversight of the care plan, either directly or indirectly, has proven beneficial to the patient's overall health.[15,16,17]

KNOWING WHEN AND WHICH HHAs OR OTHER HOME AND COMMUNITY-BASED SERVICE ORGANIZATIONS ARE WORKING WITH YOUR PATIENTS

It is impossible to play an active role in the home care plan unless you are aware that home care is being provided to a patient. Office-based physicians should insist that hospitalists inform them about home care referrals that occur at hospital discharge. Currently, there is no regulatory mandate that such information must be shared before the patient is discharged from the hospital, but it is wise to develop close relationships with the hospitalists, discharge planners and the newly developing care transitions programs to ensure that complete information about all service arrangements is available in a timely fashion (before the patient reaches home). Post-acute care home health services account for the majority of HHA referrals.[18] Referrals from the office should be documented clearly in the medical chart. Under the Patient Protection and Affordable Care Act, the primary physician has added responsibility to document a face-to-face visit with the patient in determining and authorizing Medicare home health services (see details below).

HAVING DIRECT CONTACT WITH PATIENTS RECEIVING HOME CARE

Home health nursing visits supplement primary physician care, but should not be considered a substitute for it. Patients receiving home health services should be seen at a frequency comparable to other patients with similar conditions and severity of disease. As noted above, effective April 2011 a physician who certifies a patient as eligible for Medicare home health services must see the patient. The law also allows the requirement to be satisfied if a nurse practitioner or physician assistant sees the patient, when they are working for or in collaboration with the physician. As part of the certification form itself, or as an addendum to it, they must document that they saw the patient, and document how the patient's clinical condition supports a homebound status and need for skilled services. The face-to-face encounter must occur within the 90 days prior to the start of home health care, or within the 30 days after the start of care. In a situation when a physician orders home health care for the patient based on a new condition that was not evident during a visit within the 90 days prior to the start of care, the certifying physician (or nurse practitioner or physician assistant working in collaboration with the physician) must see the patient within 30 days after admission.

Recognizing the difficulty this mandate may impose, the regulations allow some accommodations: 1) A physician who attended to the patient in an acute or post-acute setting, but does not follow the patient into the community (such as a hospitalist) is allowed to certify the need for home health care based on his or her contact with the patient, and establish and sign the plan of care. The acute/post-acute physician would then "hand-off" the patient's care to his or her community-based physician. 2) Medicare will also allow physicians who attended to the patient in an acute or post-acute setting to certify the need for home health care based on his or her contact with the patient, initiate the orders for home health services, and "hand off" the patient to his or her community-based physician to review and sign off on the plan of care. 3) The law allows the face-to-face encounter to occur via telehealth in rural areas in an approved originating site (see http://www.cms.gov/MLNMattersArticles/downloads/SE1038.pdf).

While current law and regulations require a physician to certify the need for home health services, many physicians are expanding their coverage of these complex patients with collaborative practices with advance practice clinicians (nurse practitioners or physician assistants.) As part of the 1997 Medicare Balanced Budget Act, nurse practitioners and physician assistants were given the ability to bill for services provided within their "scope of practice" regardless of site, subject to state regulations. Prior to this change, these advance practice clinicians generally needed to have their physician supervisors physically present, which discouraged their use in home visits. Examples of collaborative arrangements, sample agreements and additional information may be found through the American Academy of Home Care Physicians (see Advanced Issues in House Call Program Management, 2011, AAHCP).

COMMUNICATION AND COORDINATION OF SERVICES

Physicians who certify the need for home health care have the primary responsibility for coordinating medical care for patients receiving such care. The primary physician oversees the total care plan and must also serve as a liaison between the multiple specialists, surgeons, and others who may be involved in the patient's care. An organized system for communication with HHAs or home and community-based services can facilitate effective patient care, care plan oversight, and certification or recertification of medical necessity of the home care services.[19]

Critical communication and coordination activities for physicians in home care include:

➤ Providing or arranging for continuous, knowledgeable physician coverage: Home care patients and the home health professionals serving them need 24-hour telephone access to a primary physician. When home care involves high-technology equipment, home infusion therapy, or hospice services, it is critical that covering physicians be knowledgeable of the situation and comfortable managing complex scenarios to avoid unnecessary emergency room visits and hospitalizations for problems that can be addressed at home.

➤ Maintaining organized records of home care services: Office charts should include copies of all signed orders; evaluations and reports from home health team members; notes from telephone conversations; and names of all organizations, personnel, and consulting physicians involved in the patient's care. Given the significant amount of regulations/requirements surrounding home care services, it is critical that documentation in the medical record be accurate, accessible and complete. Medicare requires that home care certification forms be retained by the physician for seven years.

➤ Prompt response to telephone calls from HHA staff: Telephone calls should be returned the same day they are received. When a home health provider requests an urgent response, a system should be available just as it is for calls from an intensive care unit nurse or another physician. Many physicians are now choosing to use alternative means of communication such as email (secured) to increase their availability and remove communication barriers.

➤ Timely response to written communications: The paperwork sent to physicians for review and signature is important for communication regarding ongoing care; physician signatures are required for billing by the HHA and timely communication assures compliance with state, federal, and accrediting agency requirements. Laboratory reports sent from HHAs (e.g., prothrombin time) should generally be reviewed within a day of receipt. Physicians should have a system to sign and return routine correspondence at least weekly.

➤ Communication of changes in patient condition and care plan to the HHA: Home health agencies must know of all changes in the patient's overall care plan including changes in medications, upcoming medical appointments and tests, and new diagnoses. Changes in patient condition should also be communicated, especially if they might affect eligibility for reimbursement for home care (e.g., changes in a patient's ability to leave the home). After an office visit by a home health patient, information can be communicated to the HHA via a phone call or by sending progress notes to the agency.

➤ Advocate on behalf of the patient for provision of all needed services: Many health insurers require authorization for home health services. Physicians may need to communicate directly with the staff involved when the HHA's efforts to obtain such authorization fail. Under the Medicare

Prospective Payment for home health services system, agencies receive a fixed payment for all services provided. Therefore, physicians must represent the patient's interest and advocate for them with the HHA staff so that their patients will receive all needed services. (subject to eligibility rules).

➤ Coordination of care with other health professionals who are providing care in the home through organizations other than a Medicare-certified HHA. The same patient who receives services from an HHA may also be receiving services from a community-based program that provides social work, Meals on Wheels, direct care workers, transportation, etc. They may also get services from a DME (durable medical equipment) company that may include sending trained personnel into the home to teach the patient and family how to use the equipment. Finally, patients could also be receiving case management or patient care transition coaching via telephone or through home visits. Any of these individuals may identify problems and seek to notify the physician. Taking such calls during a busy office practice may present problems that can be mitigated by developing a template of questions to fully inform the physician about what is happening to the patient in the home. Physicians should ask:

  ➤ Name of caller and contact information

  ➤ What service are they providing to the patient? Under what agency?

  ➤ What is the problem? Who else have they reported the problem to already, or will in the future (who else needs to know)?

  ➤ What is their current plan of care and will the new problem change that?

Physicians should be prepared to summarize the findings reported to them for confirmation and for agreement as to the next steps for both the caller and the other individuals who may be involved in the patient's total care plan. The conversation should be documented in the patient's medical record.

THE SITE OF CARE

Perhaps the most critical role for the physicians is determining if home care is suitable for an individual patient. Care in the home may be medically appropriate for almost any acute or chronic problem; however, situations exist where medical care is necessary, but home-based care may not be appropriate. The patient's unique home, social, and family/caregiver situations play a paramount role in decisions regarding the medical necessity for home care. For example, when diagnostic tests or therapies are considered necessary but are not available in a timely manner, patients should be referred to other settings. Factors to consider in this determination are listed in Table 6.

TABLE 6 Considerations for initiating in-home care

Service can be provided in the home

➤ Person, financial, and family/community resources available

➤ Severity of illness is such that care needs can be met in a timely manner

➤ Home-based technology exists

➤ Physicians, and other home health staff can be accessed in a timely manner

➤ Meets growth and development needs

Safety

➤ The service can be provided safely in the home

➤ Difficulty in receiving proper care in the event of complication

➤ Risk to providers in making house calls

Patient autonomy

➤ Patient's desire to remain in the home

➤ Elimination of need for more restrictive environment (e.g., hospital, nursing home)

Transportation barriers

➤ Patient stressed by need for transportation to other settings

➤ Patient unable to leave home for functional reasons

Expected outcomes

➤ Improved function, compliance, and quality of life as a result of intervention

➤ Better chance of achieving expected outcomes in home than in other settings

➤ Enhance family health and socialization

Cost-effectiveness

REFERENCES

1. Department of Health and Human Services, Office of Inspector General. *The physician's role in Medicare home health 2001*. Washington, DC: Department of Health and Human Service, Office of Inspector General. (OEI-02-00-00620; 12/01) http://www.hhs.gov/oig/oei. Accessed November 2011.

2. National Transitions of Care Coalition. *Improving on Transitions of Care: How to Implement and Evaluate a Plan*. http://www.ntocc.org/Portals/0/ImplementationPlan.pdf. Accessed February 10, 2011.

3. Coleman E, Williams W. Executing high-quality care transitions: a call to do it right. *J Hospital Medicine.* 2007;2:287–290.

4. AMA Council on Scientific Affairs. Educating physicians in home health care. *JAMA.* 1991;265:769–771.

5. Department of Health and Human Services, Office of Inspector General. *The physician's role in Medicare home health 2001.* Washington, DC: Department of Health and Human Service, Office of Inspector General. (OEI-02-00-00620; 12/01) http://www.hhs.gov/oig/oei. Accessed November 2011.

6. Department of Health and Human Services, Office of Inspector General. Home health fraud, fraud and abuse in the provision of medical supplies to nursing facilities. *Federal Register.* 1995;60:40847–40851.

7. Leff B, Burton J. The future history of home care and physician house calls in the United States. *J Gerontol.* 2001;56:603–608.

8. Jette A, Smith IC, McDermit S. Quality of Medicare reimbursed home health care. *Gerontologist.* 1996;36:492–501.

9. Ramsdell JW, Swart JA, Jackson JE, Renvall M. The yield of a home visit in the assessment of geriatric patients. *J Am Geriatr Soc.* 1989;37:17–24.

10. Kravitz R, Reuben D, Davis J, et al. Geriatric home assessment after hospital discharge. *J Am Geriatr Soc.* 1994;42:1229–1234.

11. Stuck A, Aronow H, Steiner A, et al. A trial of annual in-home comprehensive geriatric assessment. *N Engl J Med.* 1995;333:1184–1189.

12. Rothkopf MM. The physician's role in home care: doctoring in a hospital without walls. In: Standards and Practice of Home Care Therapeutics. 2nd ed. Baltimore, MD: Williams and Wilkins; 1997.

13. Visanathan R, Macintosh C, Callary M, Penhall R, Horowitz M, Chapman I. The nutritional status of 250 older Australian recipients of domiciliary care services and its association with outcomes at 12 months. *J Am Geriatric Society.* 2003;51:1007–1011.

14. Peng TR, Navaie-Waliser M, Feldman PH. Social support, home health service use, and outcomes among four racial-ethnic groups. *Gerontologist.* 2003;43:503–513.

15. Melin AL, Hakansson S, Bygren LO. The cost-effectiveness of rehabilitation in the home: a study of Swedish elderly. *Am J Public Health.* 1993;83:356–362.

16. Stessman J, Ginsberg G, Hammerman-Rozenberg R, et al. Decreased hospital utilization by older adults attributable to a home hospitalization program. *J Am Geriatric Soc.* 1996;44:591–598.

17. Melin AL, Wieland D, Harker J, Bygren LO. Health outcomes of post-hospital in-home team care: secondary analysis of a Swedish trial. *J Am Geriatr Soc.* 1995;43:301–307.

18. Massachusetts Medical Society. Survey of Physician's Utilization of Home Health Services. June 2009. http://www.massmed.org. Accessed September 13, 2010.

19. Making Home Care Work In Your Practice: A Brief Guide to Reimbursement and Regulations. American Academy of Home Care Physicians, www.aahcp.org. Accessed January 2011.

CHAPTER | THREE

The Physician-Patient-Caregiver Relationship

After reading this chapter you should be able to:

1. Identify methods to effectively communicate with patients in the home care setting

2. Describe the scope of and common caregiver issues

3. Identify strategies to enhance the patient-caregiver relationship in home care

4. Identify strategies to enhance the physician-caregiver relationship in home care

Regardless of the venue, successful physician-patient relationship are built on effective clinical and communication skills, responsive and continuous care, and understanding the needs of patients. This might include specific information relevant to diagnosis, treatments, prognosis, and general health education as well as working with caregivers and coordinating care that may involve specialists, ancillary therapists and social services. This is especially true for home care patients. Patients in need of home care usually have multiple, complex medical problems that require increased assistance from the physician to understand the illnesses and what is required to manage them most effectively in home-based care. In addition to medical oversight of frequently fluctuating chronic condition(s), physicians involved in effective home care must be able to advise, encourage, and support the patient and his or her caregivers. Whether the patient is a child with severe asthma or a geriatric patient with multiple chronic problems, physician home visits can enhance understanding of the dynamic context and be a source of both professional satisfaction and maintenance of trust in the physician-patient relationship. It is imperative that the physician and others involved in home care ensure that patients and caregivers understand the issues and aims of the home care plan.

TABLE 1 Topics for effective physician-patient communication in home care

➤ Effects of disease and treatment on the patient's daily functioning and lifestyle

➤ Expected course of the illness, both short- and long-term

➤ Tasks that the patient and/or caregiver will be expected to perform

➤ Capacity of home caregiver(s) relative to the care needs

➤ Stress and burdens arising from chronic illness and methods to relieve such stress for both the patient and caregiver(s)

➤ Potential for rehabilitation

➤ Preventive care and counseling

➤ Special nutritional considerations

➤ Psychosocial needs

➤ Importance of monitoring the condition(s) by the patient and/or caregiver(s)

➤ Early signs of instability or deterioration that should be reported to the physician

➤ Improvements in function or condition that should be reported to the physician

➤ Advance directives

An ever-growing population of complex and chronically ill patients of all ages with a great diversity of medical and psychosocial needs is now being cared for in the home. The increasing focus on the Patient Centered Medical Home (PCMH) and the evolving payment paradigms that reward outcomes and/or require more cost-efficient, comprehensive care through Accountable Care Organizations (ACO) or other population-based bundling make effective home care an important part of both health systems and physician practices. This care is possible only through the trust and compliance of patients and caregivers.

CAREGIVER ISSUES

Family caregivers provide at least 80% of the care received by individuals in the community. More than 65 million people, 29% of the U.S. population, provide care for a chronically ill, disabled or aged family member or friend during any given year and spend an average of 20 hours per week providing care for their loved one. The value of family caregiver services is estimated to be $375 billion a year—almost twice as much as is spent on home care and nursing home services combined ($158 billion). The typical family caregiver is a 49-year-old woman

TABLE 2 Topics of special importance to pediatric home care patients

- ➤ Optimal nutrition and feeding
- ➤ Therapy options for rehabilitation
- ➤ Modification of technology support (for high-technology home care) for optimal function
- ➤ Educational and socialization needs
- ➤ Issues related to promotion of optimal growth and development
- ➤ Effects of chronic illness/disability on social development/sibling and/or family relations
- ➤ Family/marital stress due to parenting a child with special needs

caring for her widowed 69-year-old mother who does not live with her. She is married and employed. Approximately 66% of family caregivers are women. More than 37% have children or grandchildren under 18 years of age living with them. Family caregivers spend an average of 20 hours per week caring for their loved ones; 13% provide 40 hours or more of care per week. Fourteen percent of family caregivers care for a special needs child, with an estimated 16.8 million caring for special needs children under 18 years of age.[1]

Substantial financial burdens are associated with the caregiving role. Seventy-three percent of family caregivers who care for someone over age 18 years either work or have worked while providing care; 66% have had to make adjustments to their work life, from reporting late to giving up employment entirely; and 1 in 5 family caregivers have had to take a leave of absence. Forty-seven percent of working caregivers report that caregiving expenses have caused them to use up all or most of their savings. The average family caregiver for someone 50 years or older spent $5,531 on out-of-pocket caregiving expenses in 2007, which was more than 10% of the median income for a family caregiver that year.[1]

The difficulties of care provision and balancing caregiving with other family and employment responsibilities affect emotional health. Forty to 70% of family caregivers have clinically significant symptoms of depression and approximately 25% to 50% of these caregivers meet the diagnostic criteria for major depression.[2]

The burden of caregiving stems from a complex interaction of factors. Patient-specific factors include behavioral problems, the difficulty mastering skills required to provide treatment and maintenance regimens, and the ability or willingness of the patient to assist in care. Caregiver-specific factors include the caregiver's health, perceived competence, and commitment. Finally, the nature of the relationship and the ability of both parties to compromise and adjust to one another's needs are highly important. A self-assessment of caregiver burden and other resources are available from the American Medical Association (see

Appendix A or visit *http://www.ama-assn.org/ama/pub/physician-resources/ public-health/promoting-healthy-lifestyles/geriatric-health/caregiver-health/ caregiver-self-assessment.shtml*).

THE PATIENT-CAREGIVER RELATIONSHIP

The patient and caregiver form a unit with the dependencies of the patient matched by the capabilities and willingness of the caregiver to provide assistance and support. A comprehensive home-based approach to care should provide the full range of treatments and service resources necessary to support the patient-caregiver unit. Formal public and private agency services may supply the skills and abilities that the caregiver cannot provide.

A systematic approach to identifying the strengths and weaknesses of the patient-caregiver functional relationship is central to developing the medical care plan and provides a measurable set of goals for success. Functions most likely to respond to clinical improvements or rehabilitative efforts can be identified by matching the dependencies noted in the initial patient functional assessment to the underlying co-morbidities. This also helps identify areas of training to target to enhance the caregiver's skills. Supporting the patient-caregiver relationship is an important goal of home care and counseling programs are often available. The Older American Act and some state Medicaid programs provide support for caregiver coaching. Information on such programs is available from local Area Agencies on Aging (see Chapters 6, 7 and 17 for additional information).

Ideally, responsibility for each part of the care plan should be assigned to either the patient or the caregiver. If neither is capable in certain areas, or the caregiver is unwilling to assume certain responsibilities, then secondary caregivers may be needed. These services may be acquired through referral to a home care, social service or legal agency, or the family may wish to hire the necessary personnel directly. Periodic reassessment, especially if there are significant changes in clinical status (of either the patient or the caregiver), helps to maintain stability of the home care program. Alternatively, this approach can make clear the need to consider institutionalization. A more extensive list of factors that impact the caregiver-patient relationship along with information on how to intervene and develop a care plan can be found at http://www1.us.elsevierhealth.com/MERLIN/ Gulanick/Constructor/index.cfm?plan=10.

Physician support of caregivers is critical and multi-factorial. Caregivers often experience a sense of isolation and can be highly dependent on their relationship with the patient's physician. They see the physician as a de facto case manager who provides appropriate connections with health, social service agency, and specialty referrals to assist in clinical management. The physician should validate the caregiving role by affirming the work of caregiving and acknowledging the stress, loneliness, and burden. Caregivers and patients must be frequently assessed and reassessed to identify behavioral, functional, and physical problems that may threaten the patient-caregiver unit. A home visit provides significant emotional support to the caregiver as well as a means for continuing medical management.

Training the caregiver to recognize the specific signs and symptoms of illness in the patient and to know the appropriate response ensures the caregiver's competence and the safety and well-being of the patient. Most families are highly motivated and can be successfully trained in a wide variety of therapeutic, diagnostic, and behavioral management skills. The caregiver needs to understand that new behavioral problems should be evaluated expeditiously because these changes often signal an acute problem, such as acute delirium, requiring prompt diagnostic and therapeutic intervention. If the aberrant behavior is not based on an acute physiologic problem, specific recommendations involving either behavioral management or psychopharmacologic therapies may be provided. Physicians can also anticipate problems such as pressure sores, urinary tract infections with chronic Foley catheters and gastrostomy tube malfunctions. Appropriate instructions, durable medical equipment, urine containers/antibiotics, and replacement gastrostomy tubes can be provided in the home to avert these potential problems. Anticipating such problems can help patients and caregivers avoid the trauma and cost of emergency department visits.

Caregiver's stress or frustration are important factors associated with failure of the care plan, abuse, or premature institutionalization.[3] It is important to recognize and develop plans to deal with caregiver stress. Caregiver well-being has been shown to be affected by patient behavioral problems, frequency of caregiving breaks, self-esteem, perceived social support, burden, and hours of informal care.[4] Various interventions (e.g., respite and caregiver education) have been shown to be effective in improving patient outcomes and relieving caregiver stress[5,6,7] associated with caring for patients with dementia. The American College of Physicians has an excellent resource on the ethics of the physician-caregiver relationship (www.acponline.org/running_practice/ethics/issues/policy/caregivers.pdf).

RESOURCES

Parent caregiver support: National Family Caregiver Alliance: www.nfcacares.org

National Center on Caregiving: www.caregiver.org

REFERENCES

1. Caregiving Statistics. National Family Caregivers Association web site. http://www
.nfcacares.org/who_are_family_caregivers/care_giving_statstics.cfm. Accessed
September 19, 2011.

2. Zarit S. Assessment of family caregivers: A research perspective. In: Family Caregiver
Alliance (eds), Caregiver Assessment: Voices and Views from the Field. Report from a
National Consensus Development Conference. Vol. II, pp. 12–37. San Francisco: Family
Caregiver Alliance; 2006.

3. Shugarman LR, Buttar A, Fries BE, Moore T, Blaum CS. Caregiver attitudes and
hospitalization risk in Michigan residents receiving home- and community-based care.
J Am Geriatr Soc. 2002;50:1079–1085.

4. Chappell NL, Reid RC. Burden and well-being among caregivers: examining the distinction.
Gerontologist. 2002;42:772–780.

5. Grant I, McKibbin CL, Taylor MJ, Mills P, Dimsdale J, Ziegler M, Patterson TL. In-home
respite intervention reduces plasma epinephrine in stressed Alzheimer caregivers. *Am J
Geriatr Psychiatry.* 2003;11:62–72.

6. Hebert R, Levesque L, Vezina J, Lavoie JP, Ducharme F, Gendron C, Preville M, Voyer L,
Dubois MF. Efficacy of a psychoeducative group program for caregivers of demented
persons living at home: a randomized controlled trial. *J Gerontol B Psychol Sci Soc Sci.*
2003;58:S58–S67.

7. Brodaty H, Green A, Koschera A. Meta-analysis of psychosocial interventions for caregivers
of people with dementia. *J Am Geriatr Soc.* 2003;51:657–664.

CHAPTER FOUR

Eligibility and Coverage for Home Care Services

After reading this chapter you should be able to:

1. Describe the physician's responsibility in development and oversight of the home care plan

2. Describe the factors affecting the frequency and duration of home care services

3. Explain homebound status documentation according to Medicare's definition of eligibility for skilled home care services

4. Select appropriate Medicare-covered home health services for referral

Medicare and other payers reimburse for home-based health care under multiple types of health insurance benefits. Skilled home care is generally limited to patients who are considered homebound, although non-Medicare providers waive this requirement for patients receiving home infusion services. It is not necessary to be homebound to receive home-based rehabilitation under Medicare's outpatient rehabilitation benefit, hospice under hospice benefits, or medical care in the home (provided by physicians, nurse practitioners, and physician assistants). Insurers do not require patients to be homebound to receive durable medical equipment such as wheelchairs or oxygen. In all cases, however, physicians must certify the need for the care, often subject to insurers' guidelines for medical necessity and eligibility. Co-pays and deductibles vary across these types of insurance benefits and by insurer.

PHYSICIAN RESPONSIBILITIES

The prescribing physician is responsible for the initiation and ongoing review of home care funded by Medicare and most other payers, and must clearly define the purpose of providing skilled home health care services in the plan of care.[1] This involves choosing the treatments and services that are appropriate and medically necessary to reach desired treatment outcomes, knowing which services can be provided by individual members of the home health staff, and projecting the frequency and duration of those services needed to reach the defined outcomes. The amount of care the patient requires is determined by the acuity of his or her condition, the level of skilled care the patient needs, and the level of technology needed.

The Medicare home health benefit will cover skilled services when the care is such that it could only be performed safely by a skilled professional. The development and oversight of the treatment plan is the responsibility of the prescribing physician, is supervised by the skilled professionals (e.g., registered nurse, physical therapist, speech therapist), and carried out by these professionals and an extended home care team including home health aides and family caregivers. For patients to be eligible for Medicare-reimbursed skilled home health care, there must be a reasonable probability of improvement in the problem being treated. In some cases, determining the potential for wound healing or meaningful rehabilitation may require input from a vascular surgeon or physician specializing in rehabilitation medicine, respectively.

The prescribing physician must determine the scope and frequency of home care services when developing and reviewing the care plan. A patient's nursing and other home care needs depend on his or her medical problems and abilities, and also the abilities and willingness of caregivers to learn and carry out the delegated nursing tasks (such as dressing changes). Some patients with multiple complex morbidities are essentially chronically unstable and require both physician and nursing interventions on a periodic basis.

If physician home visits are offered, the frequency of these visits will also vary depending on the patient's co-morbidities, the relative risk-versus-benefit of aggressive therapies, the need for documentation in the noncompliant caregiver situation, or the instability of both social and medical factors (see Table 1). As is the case with physicians' services in the office, the scope, frequency, and duration of home care is highly individual and is determined by the patient's needs and resources. Some Medicare carriers have guidelines that limit reimbursement for physician home visits when patients are also receiving skilled home care. Since home health agencies (HHA) are paid prospectively for all their visits, physicians must provide a service that could not have been provided by the home care nurse. For example, a physician visit simply to observe a wound and change a dressing or to check blood pressure management could fail to meet an auditor's criteria.

TABLE 1 Factors determining frequency of home care services

➤ Acuity/instability of illness, need for observation and intervention

➤ Complexity of treatment prescribed

➤ Patient and/or caregiver need for education to learn how to safely provide the prescribed treatment

➤ Patient or caregiver need for psychosocial support to manage the treatment at home

These distinctions are described by one Medicare carrier in a local coverage decision WPS Medicare Local Coverage Decision phys081 (www.wpsmedicare .com/part_b/policy/active/local/131613_phys081.shtml), stating that services provided in the home or domiciliary setting must not unnecessarily duplicate services provided to the beneficiary by other practitioners, regardless of whether those practitioners provide the service in the office, facility or home/domiciliary setting. Home/domiciliary services provided for the same diagnosis, same condition or same episode of care as services provided by other practitioners, regardless of the site of service, may constitute concurrent or duplicative care. When such services are provided, the record must clearly document the medical necessity of such services. When documentation is lacking, the service may be considered not medically necessary. The evaluation and management (E/M) service will not be considered medically necessary when it is performed only to provide supervision for a visiting nurse or HHA visit(s).

The patient and caregivers should view the physician and practice staff as a critical resource in understanding and advising on options and funding of home care in the face of acute and chronic illness. These options may include long-term-care insurance, government programs such as In-Home Support Services and Home and Community-Based Services (These home-based programs vary by state. To learn about a particular state's programs and for contact information see Chapter 17 for the list of state agencies. State laws or payers' policies may require a physician's declaration of mental competence or a written evaluation of the safety of a given patient living in the community. Physicians also need to consider the risks of elder abuse, especially financial elder abuse, in supporting the final decision for a patient to stay at home. These issues become quite complex and may require several home visits with care coordination involving appropriate authorities, such as adult protective services, before an appropriate disposition can be made.

The duration of home care services should depend on achievement of the care plan's predetermined, expected outcomes (see Table 2). Outcomes may be straightforward and easily documented (e.g., healing progress of a wound or improvement with physical therapy) or more difficult to quantify such as simply avoiding institutional care. The physician may wish to make a house call before discharging a patient from home care.

TABLE 2 Factors affecting the duration of home care services

➤ Achievement of expected goals and outcomes of care

➤ Overall prognosis

➤ Unanticipated complications from expected outcomes

➤ Need for continuing skilled services because of inability of patient or caregiver to evaluate and provide appropriate care independently

MEDICAL NECESSITY

Medical necessity is a critical element of Medicare and most other types of insurance coverage. What constitutes medically necessary care has not been determined in a scientific manner. Some aspects of medical necessity apply regardless of the site of care (Table 3). Medical necessity determinations are typically based on a combination of acuity of the illness/injury, patient comorbidity, and patient dependency. Other models of medical necessity

TABLE 3 Considerations for the determination of medical necessity in any setting

Acuity/severity of illness

➤ Physiologic abnormalities

➤ Uncontrolled symptoms

➤ Risk of adverse events

➤ Frequency of clinical judgments/re-evaluations

Comorbidities

➤ Interrelationships of multiple disease processes and multiple treatments

➤ Medical complexity

Dependency

➤ Functional impairments caused by disease(s) may require:

    ➤ Equipment and training in its use

    ➤ Assistance of another person (skilled or unskilled)

    ➤ Education for self care

    ➤ Rehabilitative therapy

    ➤ Prevention of excess disability/risk management

emphasize prognosis and obtainable outcomes. For pediatric patients, the American Academy of Pediatrics includes in its definition of medical necessity not only the outcomes the service will have on the patient's condition, illness, or injury, but also questions of the age appropriateness of services, their effect on mental and physical growth, and the maintenance of functional capacity.[2]

MEDICARE HOME HEALTH CARE

Medicare Home Health Care is defined as "skilled nursing care and certain other health services provided in a person's home to treat an illness or injury."[3] Medicare will pay for home health care if it is medically necessary for treating a person's illness or injury. Medicare has specific guidelines for beneficiaries to qualify for Medicare Home Health Care and certain criteria for the services covered. A useful resource is the American Academy of Home Care Physicians' *Making Home Care Work in a Medical Practice*.

HOMEBOUND STATUS

The definition of homebound may not be an issue for patients who pay for the services themselves, but it is when considering eligibility for payment of home care services by Medicare and some other insurers. The beneficiary must be homebound to be eligible for the Medicare Home Health Care coverage. A patient is considered homebound if "leaving the home would require a considerable and taxing effort" and if the patient "has a condition due to illness or injury which restricts ability to leave the residence except with the aid of supportive devices, the use of special transportation, or the assistance of another person, or if the patient has a condition such that leaving the home is medically contraindicated." Homebound patients may leave the home "if absences are infrequent or for periods of relatively short duration...or for the purpose of receiving medical treatment." Participation in adult day services is permissible under this definition of homebound.[4] Physicians considering homebound status need only consider the patient's condition while receiving home care, not prior status. Thus, a patient who has been driving to social occasions daily can become suddenly homebound due to acute illness or injury. For example, almost any patient presenting to a physician with symptoms of pneumonia would be homebound temporarily and be eligible for Medicare-reimbursed home care to assist in management of symptoms or monitoring of response and tolerance to antibiotic therapy.

PLAN OF CARE

Medicare also requires that the beneficiary be under a physician's care, have a written plan of care approved by the responsible physician (defined as a licensed MD, DO or podiatrist), and need at least one of the following intermittent services: skilled nursing care, physical therapy, speech therapy, or continued occupational therapy. By itself occupational therapy does not constitute a skilled service that justifies starting skilled home care. However, after care has begun and other skilled services are discontinued, continued occupational therapy does qualify as a skilled need. Finally, the HHA must be Medicare-certified. Effective April 2011 a physician who certifies a patient as eligible for Medicare home health services must see the patient face to face and document how the patient's clinical condition supports a homebound status and the need for skilled services (see Chapter 2 and http://www.cms.gov/MLNMattersArticles/downloads/SE1038.pdf).

If the threshold coverage criteria are met, beneficiaries are entitled to receive clearly defined services as reviewed in Table 4. The beneficiary is not responsible for any deductibles or co-payments. Medicare pays the full approved cost of all covered home health visits and will pay 80% of the approved amount for certain pieces of medical equipment. Medicare does not limit the length of coverage. The physician's plan of care covers a 60-day period, or what is known as a home health benefit period. If a beneficiary requires more time, a physician must recertify that the beneficiary requires the services and continues to meet Medicare's requirements in order for Medicare to continue paying for home health care. Additional physician face-to-face encounters are not required for recertification.

Medicare does, however, limit the number of hours per day and days per week a beneficiary can receive home health services. The part-time/intermittent criteria are used both as eligibility criterion and to determine the amount of services. In determining whether an individual is eligible for home health services, Medicare defines "intermittent" skilled care as fewer than seven days a week or less than eight hours each day for a period of 21 days. Once the beneficiary is receiving home health services, Medicare limits the amount of skilled care and home health aide services to a combined total of less than eight hours per day and 28 or fewer hours each week. These limits predate the prospective payment system. Currently, these limits are rarely relevant or enforced, as Medicare-certified HHAs are unlikely to offer more than daily visits by a nurse or more than several visits per week by a therapist or home health aide. Patients receiving continuous home care services from non-Medicare community-based programs are routinely permitted to obtain Medicare-reimbursed intermittent services. This is most obvious in assisted living facilities, which did not exist when Congress wrote the Medicare laws describing eligibility.

If a beneficiary is in a private Medicare plan, such as a capitated Medicare Advantage plan, then he or she generally must use an HHA that has a contract with the HMO. Some plans require prior authorization for home care services. If the beneficiary is in the Medicare Private Fee-for-Service (PFFS) plan, then he or she can use any Medicare-certified HHA that will accept the patient. The HHA may either accept the PFFS plan's terms of payment or collect the Medicare prospective payment as if the patient were in traditional Medicare.

TABLE 4 Medicare-covered services

Skilled nursing

Some situations that might warrant skilled nursing services are:

➤ Observation and assessment of the patient's condition that can be performed safely and accurately only by a skilled professional

➤ Procedures or services that can be performed safely and effectively only by a skilled professional (e.g., intravenous fluids/drugs, intramuscular injections, Foley catheter changes)

➤ Evaluation or management of the patient care plan (including intermittent monitoring of the physiologic status of patients requiring high-technology care)

➤ Patient education (e.g., medication management, tube feedings, wound management), teaching self-care strategies (e.g., disease management such as diabetic care, congestive heart failure care)

Skilled therapy services

Medicare covers two types of therapeutic programs:

➤ Restorative therapy—provided with the expectation that the patient will improve (and such improvement can be measured) in a reasonable and generally predictable amount of time

➤ Maintenance therapy—provided with the expectation that these services are necessary for the establishment of a safe and effective maintenance program, and that the beneficiary or caregivers will be instructed and supervised in carrying it out

Specific conditions that may be amenable to therapeutic exercises; treatments; training in compensatory techniques to improve level of independence, or training in the use of assistive devices, which include but are not limited to:

➤ Loss or restriction of mobility affecting ambulation, balance, positioning, transferring, bed mobility, generalized weakness, or fatigue

➤ Loss or restriction of mobility that limits performance of activities of daily living (ADLs) (bathing, toileting, dressing, transferring, and feeding)

➤ Communication disabilities such as expressive or receptive aphasia, voice disorders, or limitations in reading or writing

➤ Swallowing difficulties

➤ Safety risk—fall prevention, training in awareness of hazards, and prevention of injury for those with functional impairments

(Continued)

TABLE 4 *Continued*

Home health aide services

When a qualifying skilled service is provided, home health aides can perform part-time and intermittent services such as:

➤ Personal care (assistance with bathing, dressing, toileting, transferring, and eating)

➤ Simple dressing changes that do not require the skills of a licensed nurse

➤ Assistance with self-administered medications that do not require the skills of a licensed nurse

➤ Assistance with therapeutic exercises that do not require the presence of a skilled therapist

➤ Routine care of prosthetic or orthotic devices

Medical social services

When a qualifying skilled service is provided, the services of a medical social worker can be covered if those services are necessary to resolve social or emotional problems that are an "impediment to the effective treatment of the patient's medical condition or rate of recovery."

Such medical social services include but are not limited to:

➤ Assessment of pertinent psychosocial and economic factors

➤ Appropriate action to obtain community resources to help the patient

➤ Counseling services for the patient

➤ Short-term counseling services (two to three visits) for family caregivers

Source: *Medicare Benefit and Policy Manual Chapter 7-Home Health Services.* www.cms.gov/manuals/Downloads/bp102c07.pdf

MEDICAID

Eligibility for Medicaid home health programs, funded jointly by state and federal governments, varies from state to state in terms of qualifying income levels and welfare status. States also vary in their coverage of services. Most programs cover part-time nursing and aide services, medical equipment, and supplies. They may or may not cover physical, speech, or occupational therapy. Some states require pre-approval before services can be provided.

In addition to traditional Medicaid skilled home health coverage, some states operate a Medicaid waiver program that enables them to provide Medicaid payments for home and community-based services to individuals who would otherwise receive Medicaid-reimbursed care in nursing homes. States must show that the home care program is more cost-effective than institutional care. Eligibility is often based on issues of dependency in ADLs or cognitive impairment. Not all states participate in Medicaid waiver programs, and localities within a state may differ in the services (e.g., qualifications and training of staff, type, frequency, and duration of services) that are covered.[5,6] Finally, some states participate in Money Follows the Person (MFP) Rebalancing Demonstration Program grants.[6] The MFP Rebalancing Demonstration Program was authorized by Congress in section 6071 of the Deficit Reduction Act of 2005 (DRA) and was designed to provide assistance to states to balance their long-term care systems and help Medicaid enrollees transition from institutions to the community. Monies that were being used to pay for institutional care are used instead for home and community-based services.[7] With this development and the pressure on budgets, state departments on aging will increasingly be held accountable for outcomes and costs and will seek vendors who can demonstrate value.

COMMERCIAL INSURANCE AND MANAGED CARE PROGRAMS

Medicare managed care organizations must provide the same home care benefits that would be allowed to a patient enrolled in fee-for-service Medicare. If a physician believes that home-based services are necessary and the type and frequency of services are within Medicare benefit limits, the managed care organizations must authorize and pay for the services or must provide the patient with a denial letter along with information about the appeal process. Most plans and programs cover some home care services; their eligibility requirements, benefits, and limitations (e.g., deductible, coinsurance, type or amount of service) vary widely. Many plans follow some or all of the Medicare guidelines but frequently limit the number of visits allowed. Some programs, such as Medicare Advantage Plans, are developing community-based care management programs based on the most cost-effective setting to provide care. These innovative programs may be more liberal in eligibility or coverage than traditional Medicare guidelines of homebound status and intermittent or part-time care and place their emphasis on clinical outcomes and cost.

PRIVATE LONG-TERM-CARE INSURANCE

Long-term-care insurance can cover a variety of home-based services. Often, the patient can be reimbursed by the insurer up to a maximum per day for services not covered by other health insurance. Eligibility for the benefits varies by policy and usually relies on functional impairment and cognitive impairment measures. The most commonly used functional impairment measure is the need for assistance or supervision in two or more ADLs (number and descriptions vary) expected to last at least 90 days. Clinical evidence or standardized testing such as the Mini-Mental State Examination are used as a measure of cognitive impairment. Coverage may be restricted by cost, type, frequency, and duration of services.

PROLONGED HOME CARE SERVICES

For many patients, there are continuing long-term-care needs when the patient cannot regain his or her independence and must rely, at least in part, on outside help. Medicare Part A rules for 60-day home health coverage periods may limit the patient's access to care. Medicare pays only for the acute home health benefit and does not cover custodial or prolonged care unless medically justified. Since there is no cap on the number or length of physician services, the use of home visits by the physician to provide medical evaluations in the absence of home health benefits may be appropriate under Medicare Part B rules, as long as such visits are medically reasonable and necessary.

Some home care patients with continuing skilled monitoring needs may be eligible for Medicare coverage. If the patient meets the criteria described in the "Management and Evaluation of the Patient Care Plan" section of the Centers for Medicare & Medicaid Services *Home Health Agency Manual* (Table 5), he or she can continue to receive Medicare-covered home health services including the skilled nursing and aide services. Patients receiving this benefit must be frequently re-evaluated and their ongoing eligibility documented.

Common examples of persons eligible for prolonged care are patients with urinary catheters requiring monthly changes or patients on monthly intramuscular vitamin B12 injections. Although skilled nursing is only required monthly,

TABLE 5 Medicare criteria for prolonged care

➤ "Underlying conditions or complications such that only a skilled nurse can ensure that essential non-skilled care is achieving its purpose, or...

➤ The complexity of the unskilled services that are a necessary part of the treatment must require the involvement of a registered nurse to promote the patient's recovery and safety in view of the patient's overall condition" patients are eligible for home health aide services for assistance with custodial care. Typically, this is limited to assistance with bathing one or twice per week even though the Medicare benefit does allow such visits much more frequently. Of note, venipuncture for the purposes of obtaining a blood sample cannot be the sole reason for Medicare home health eligibility. However, if a beneficiary qualifies for home health eligibility based on a skilled need other than venipuncture alone (e.g., eligibility based on the skilled nursing service of wound care and meets all other Medicare home health eligibility criteria), medically reasonable and necessary venipuncture coverage may continue during the 60-day episode under a home health plan of care.[3] Referrals are appropriate for Medicare-covered home health care for conditions that require venipuncture as part of the nursing evaluation, such as acute infection (e.g., complete blood count) or dehydration (electrolytes and renal function). This rule was implemented primarily to exclude from coverage ongoing eligibility based on need for monitoring of a stable dose of warfarin or thyroid replacement.

For those patients who cannot regain their independence, services may not be covered. Custodial or unskilled services that are necessary to maintain the patient at the optimum level of well-being and function are not covered by the Medicare home health benefit. Private insurance, long-term-care insurance, Medicaid, and state and local community programs may provide some coverage for these patients. The majority of unskilled services are paid for by the patient and family.

The physician's role in these cases is to refer to social services for help identifying whatever resources are available (see Chapter 7, Case management: Making use of community resources) to counsel the patient and family, and to initiate discharge planning from Medicare home health services when no further skilled services are needed.

PHYSICIAN REIMBURSEMENT FOR HOME CARE-RELATED ACTIVITIES

Physician oversight of home health care has been shown to improve outcomes and reduce hospitalization and is generally reimbursable. Understanding how to bill for such activities will permit physicians to be compensated for the additional time and effort associated with ordering and overseeing HHA services or performing home visits.[4] The basics of coding and billing are reviewed in Table 6. A good reference for coding and billing issues is the American Academy of Home Care Physicians' *Making Home Care Work in a Medical Practice: A Brief Guide to Reimbursement and Regulations.*[3]

TABLE 6 How home care activities are coded and billed

Certification and recertification of skilled home health services
➤ Medicare has created a Healthcare Common Procedure Coding System (HCPCS) code to compensate physicians for the activities related to the review, sign (by hand or electronic but not stamped) and return certification and recertification paperwork (formally called Form 485 (described in Chapter 5).
Care plan oversight
➤ Almost all insurers reimburse for time spent completing paperwork and communicating about home health patients. Typically, such reimbursement requires more than 30 minutes in a calendar month to be dedicated to these activities. Coding and documentation requirements vary by payer. Medicare currently uses HCPCS codes, while other payers use Current Procedural Terminology (CPT®) codes.
Discharge planning
➤ Hospital and nursing home evaluation and management (E/M) CPT codes have specific codes for the discharge day. Work related to referral to an HHA is included in the values of those codes.
Office visits
➤ Review of home health records and communication with family or HHA staff that is part of a patient's office visit should be documented and considered in determining the complexity of decision-making, which helps determine the most appropriate CPT code for the visit.
Home visits
➤ There is a family of CPT codes specifically for physician home visits. Office-based codes should not be used for home visits. Reimbursement for home visits is generally higher than for comparable office visits, in part because of the additional types of assessments that are performed in the home. "Home" versus "domiciliary care" or "nursing home" has been defined by Medicare.
➤ Current codes, code descriptions, and values can be found on the American Academy of Home Care Physicians Web site (www.aahcp.org).

PAPERWORK RELATED TO HOME CARE

Medical services related to care in the home create a wide variety of paperwork, primarily to satisfy payers' requirements. Physician signatures are required on many documents, for both medical and non-medical purposes. Table 7 provides a list of many such forms, some of which may be state specific.

TABLE 7 Forms and documents for physician review and/or signature related to home care

Form/document	Type of service
Certification and plan of care (formerly called Form 485)	Home health care from Medicare- or Medicaid-certified agency
Attestation of face-to-face visit for Medicare skilled care	Medicare-reimbursed home care
Certificate of medical necessity	Durable medical equipment
Verbal orders	All types of home care nursing, therapies, etc
Verification of need for home care	Personal care attendant services reimbursed by Medicaid
Need for alternative payee	Social Security
Verification of disability	Long-term care benefits, need for additional key (for caregiver) in public housing
Verification of last visit date	Waiver of coroner investigation for home death
Physician order for life-sustaining treatment	Limitation in care at end of life
Hospice certification of life expectancy	Hospice care reimbursed by Medicare
Laboratory reports	Various
Missed home care visit notification	Skilled home care
Home care professionals' assessments	Various
Hospice interdisciplinary team notes	Hospice
Discharge summaries	Various
Death certificate	Various

RESOURCES

CMS Medicare and Home Health Care: http://www.medicare.gov/publications/pubs/pdf/10969.pdf

Medicare Benefit and Policy Manual Chapter 7-Home Health Services. www.cms.gov/manuals/ Downloads/bp102c07.pdf

American Academy of Home Care Physicians' *Making Home Care Work in a Medical Practice* (Revised February 2011, contact AAHCP (410) 676-7966 or www.aahcp.org).

REFERENCES

1. Centers for Medicare & Medicaid Services. *Home Health Agency Manual,* section 204.2. Baltimore, MD: Centers for Medicare & Medicaid Services. https://www.cms.gov/transmittals/downloads/R298HHA.pdf. Accessed September 20, 2011.

2. Berman S. A pediatric perspective on medical necessity. *Arch Pediatr Adolesc Med.* 1997;151:858–859.

3. American Academy of Home Care Physicians. *Making Home Care Work in a Medical Practice.* Edgewood, MD: American Academy of Home Care Physicians; 2011.

4. Centers for Medicare & Medicaid Services. *Medicare Benefit and Policy Manual Chapter 7-Home Health Services. 301.1-Patient confined to Home.* Baltimore, MD: Centers for Medicare & Medicaid Services. www.cms.gov/manuals/Downloads/bp102c07.pdf. Accessed September 20, 2011.

5. Centers for Medicare & Medicaid Services. *CMS HCBS (Home and Community Based Services) Waivers-Section 1915 (c).* Baltimore, MD: Centers for Medicare & Medicaid Services. www.cms.gov/MedicaidStWaivProgDemoPGI/05_HCBSWaivers-Section1915(c).asp. Accessed September 20, 2011.

6. The Clearinghouse for Home and Community Based Services web site. www.hcbs.org. Accessed September 20, 2011.

7. Centers for Medicare and Medicaid Services Money Follows the Person web site. https://www.cms.gov/CommunityServices/20_MFP.asp. Accessed September 20, 2011.

CHAPTER FIVE

Implementation and Oversight of the Home Care Plan

After reading this chapter you should be able to:

1. Describe the physician's role in the initiation and management of home care

2. Explain how to collaboratively develop a home health care plan and its key elements

3. Detect when home care may not be appropriate and identify alternatives for care

4. Identify strategies to effectively function as part of an interdisciplinary team in home care

The physician initiating home care plays the central role in managing the patient's in-home care. When referring a patient to a home health agency (HHA), the physician must develop and/or approve the care plan. Ongoing oversight of home care services is then required by that physician or by another physician, nurse practitioner, or physician assistant identified by the referring physician. This oversight involves collaboration and communication between the referring physician and a variety of others participating in the care of the patient.

The initial referral may occur in the course of hospital discharge planning or may be initiated from the home or clinic. The referral is usually made by directly contacting an HHA representative or through referral to a facility-based discharge planner, case manager or community-based nurse or social worker.

When referring a Medicare patient to an HHA, that agency must be Medicare-certified and the patient must meet the Centers for Medicare & Medicaid Services' definition of "homebound" if Medicare is to provide payment.

For third-party insurers, the referring physician must attest to medical necessity for home care for the services to be reimbursed. Effective April 2011 a physician who certifies a patient as eligible for Medicare home health services must see the patient face to face and document how the patient's clinical condition supports a homebound status and the need for skilled services (see Chapter 2 and http://www.cms.gov/MLNMattersArticles/downloads/SE1038.pdf). For some services (e.g., 24-hour personal attendant), it is necessary for the patient to provide payment. It is important for the referring physician and family to clearly understand the terms and cost of such care.

Patients discharged to home from the hospital or after a short-term nursing home stay often have ongoing needs for nursing, rehabilitation, or custodial care. Care planning should anticipate these needs before discharge to ensure timely initiation of the appropriate services and delivery of needed equipment. The hospital discharge planner or nursing home social worker will usually work with the patient and family in selecting an HHA in these settings. An interested physician can be involved in this process, but the physician's usual responsibility is determining the scope of home care. See Table 1 for a summary of the physician's role in the initiation and management of home care.

Children may require special considerations in this process (Table 2).

As outpatient care becomes increasingly complex, many patients require home health services without a preceding hospitalization. Physicians must be able to refer to an HHA or other community resources without the assistance of an institution's discharge planner. Some HHAs will provide referral forms similar

TABLE 1 The physician's role in the initiation and management of home care

➤ Consider the feasibility of the home as an alternative setting of care upon admission to the hospital or nursing home and reassess this frequently.

➤ Collaborate with nursing and social work staff to plan for post-discharge home-based care beginning early in the hospital stay.

➤ Clarify which physician(s) will be responsible for oversight of post-discharge care on all discharge forms, including home health referral forms. Inform the patient and caregivers how/when/whom to contact for specific problems and when follow-up appointments are or should be scheduled.

➤ Participate in the choice of an HHA to ensure that the patient's right to choose is maintained and that the agency selected can provide the services the patient requires in a timely and appropriate manner.

➤ Consider the appropriateness of the housing for the patient's types of disabilities and needs (e.g., handicapped accessibility issues).

➤ Consider the informal caregivers' (family, neighbors) capacities to help the patient and their needs for respite or training.

➤ When home health care is required, prepare a clear prescription for initial home care needs, including disciplines to be involved (e.g., nursing, therapies, social work), special assessments desired (e.g., orthostatic blood pressures, laboratory tests), and treatments required (e.g., wound dressings).

➤ Complete prescriptions for all new medications, for refills for medications that may have run out, and any equipment that is needed to permit discharge (e.g., hospital bed, wheelchair).

➤ Prepare documentation summarizing the inpatient/nursing home stay for the HHA. Ideally, a discharge summary can be sent home with the patient or faxed to the HHA at the time of discharge.

➤ Participate in patient/caregiver education related to medications, self-management strategies for the patient's illness, and expected course of illness.

TABLE 2 Additional physician responsibilities when caring for children with chronic illness disability

➤ Assess school-based and community options for health care and promotion of optimal development (e.g., early intervention programs).

➤ Understand and help coordinate the multiple care plans created by home health care providers, medical equipment vendors, early intervention programs, schools, and government and insurance company case managers.

➤ When school-aged children are technology-dependent, ensure that school staff and environment are adequate to meet the child's needs.

to those used in hospitals to simplify the documentation process. Throughout the course of the home care episode, the referring physician is responsible for reviewing the care and completing the paperwork. These activities are reimbursed in some cases (see Chapter 4, Table 6).

THE CARE PLAN

When an HHA initiates care, a written care plan is developed. The care plan is developed in a collaborative process between the HHA staff and the attending physician. Recertification is generally required every 60 days on the same form. The care plan is based on a comprehensive assessment of the patient, the home, and the availability of other caregivers. The patient's third-party insurance coverage for home care services and his or her ability to pay for needed services not covered by insurance should also be considered. Specific services rendered by physical, speech, and occupational therapists may involve different modalities. Modalities usually mentioned are for heat, ultrasound, cold, and electronic stimulation. Instructions defining the amount or duration of each modality are necessary when a discipline is providing a specific modality for therapy (e.g., PT – To apply hot packs to the C5-C6 x 10 minutes 3x/wk x 2 wks).

Example of a physician's orders	
➤ OT – Eval., ADL training, fine motor coordination	3x/wk x 6 wks
➤ ST – Eval., speech articulation disorder treatment	3x/wk x 4 wks
➤ SN – Skilled observation and assessment (e.g., cardio-pulmonary/neuro status), instruct meds, diet, hydration, etc.	3x/wk x 2 wks
➤ AIDE – Assist with personal care, catheter care	3x/wk x 9 wks

PRN visits may be ordered on a plan of care only where they are qualified in a manner that is specific to the patient's potential needs. Both the nature of the services and the number of PRN visits to be permitted for each type of service must be specified on the order form. Open-ended, unqualified PRN visits are not acceptable. A home care plan should also include specific treatment goals and a realistic evaluation of rehabilitation potential. This can serve as the basis for the development of an effective discharge plan.

Example of an appropriate PRN order

➤ Skilled nursing visits 1 x m x 2m for Foley change and PRN x 2 for emergency Foley irrigations and/or changes

➤ Skilled nursing visits 1 x m x 2m to draw blood sugar and PRN x 2 to draw emergency blood sugar if blood sugar level is above 400

Example of realistic goals

➤ Independence in transfers and ambulation with walker

➤ Healing of leg ulcer(s)

➤ Maintain patency of Foley catheter; decrease risk of urinary infection

➤ Achieve optimal level of cardiovascular status

➤ Medication and diet compliance

➤ Ability to demonstrate correct insulin preparation and administration

The physician must sign the care plan certifying the need for the home care prescribed and attesting to the patient's status as being homebound. Centers for Medicare & Medicaid Services (CMS) form 485 (the Home Health Certification and Plan of Care) meets regulatory and national survey requirements for physician plan of care certification and recertification (see www.cms.gov/trans-mittals/downloads/R23PIM.pdf). However, HHAs may submit any document that is signed and dated by the physician that contains all the required data elements. Several sources call this form, which can use the 485 format or any other that has the required elements, the "Home Health Certification and Care Plan." There are federal penalties for falsely completing this certification when Medicare is paying for the home care.

In addition to the certification form, HHAs typically have more detailed care plans for use in communicating between professionals within the agency. The roles and tasks of each professional at each visit are described. In addition, these

TABLE 3 Key elements of certification

➤ Patient demographics

➤ When home health care was initiated (start of care)

➤ The 60-day period for which the plan is being used

➤ The home care provider's name and provider number

➤ Medications: dose/frequency/route

➤ Diagnoses and surgical procedures

➤ Durable medical equipment and supplies that are separately billable

➤ Safety measures ordered by the physician

➤ Physician's order for the diet, including specific therapeutic diets and/or any specific dietary requirements; record of fluid needs or restrictions and administration of total parenteral nutrition (TPN)

➤ Allergies to medications, food, or supplies (e.g., adhesive tape, latex)

➤ Functional limitations

➤ Activities permitted

➤ Mental status

➤ Prognosis (e.g., poor, guarded, fair, good, or excellent)

➤ Orders for the amount, frequency, and duration of visits for each discipline that will be involved in home care, including duties and treatments; disciplines include skilled nursing (SN), physical therapy (PT), speech therapy (ST), occupational therapy (OT), social work (SW), or home health aide (AIDE) care plans should describe the roles of the patient, family members, or other people in the home who participate in the care plan. In some agencies, pathways for care for common diagnoses are developed.

ALTERNATIVES TO HOME CARE

The initiation or continuation of home care is not always appropriate (Table 4). The emotional and physical well-being of the caregiver, the safety of others in the home, and the willingness of the patient to participate as a partner in the home care plan are critical at all stages of home care.

The decision not to initiate or to terminate home care requires the physician to offer another care strategy (Table 5) while continuing to provide medical management throughout the patient's course of illness (unless discharged by the patient). The physician may not discontinue patient care if further treatment is

TABLE 4 Home care may not be appropriate when:

➤ Goals of treatment have been reached and the patient and caregiver(s) are independent in providing care.

➤ Changes in the course of illness or the required treatment make the home an inappropriate site for care

➤ Patient or caregiver refuses to continue home care

➤ Patient is not responsive to home care interventions

➤ Caregiver burnout and inability to obtain alternate caregiver is evident

➤ There is evidence of patient abuse or neglect that has not responded to home care interventions

➤ Gross noncompliance is identified

➤ Safety of patient or provider is threatened

➤ Irresolvable problems persist between patient/caregiver and home care team

TABLE 5 Other care settings or strategies may include the following:

➤ Acute or chronic care hospital

➤ Outpatient services/clinic programs

➤ Nursing homes

➤ Continuing care facility (board and care, life care community, licensed adult home)

➤ Adult day care/PACE (Program of All Inclusive Care for the Elderly)

➤ Medical day care for children with special needs

➤ Other family care options

➤ Group home with shared services, assisted living facility

➤ Foster homes

➤ Respite care

➤ Residential hospice care

medically indicated unless provision is made for an alternative physician or the patient refuses all further treatment.

THE INTERDISCIPLINARY TEAM

A unique aspect of home health care is the nature of the collaborative team effort. Team members must be carefully chosen to fill the needed roles and services necessary for optimal patient care. Unlike most other health care teams, home health professionals, including the attending physician, have roles that typically overlap in a set of shared tasks. This model has developed because unlike in hospitals, each professional cannot visit the patient daily and services are intermittent and not available around the clock. Knowing the expectations and limitations of each service can help ensure that the appropriate members are on the team. At each home visit and during every physician encounter, the following four tasks should be performed regardless of the professional discipline involved (Table 6).

TABLE 6 Review of interdisciplinary team and coordination of care

At each home visit and during every physician encounter, the following four tasks should be performed regardless of professional discipline involved:
➤ Assessment of the overall effectiveness of the comprehensive home care program
➤ Assessment of interactions between the patient and informal caregivers and their satisfaction with the home care program
➤ Identification, documentation, and communication to appropriate team members of any new problems and needed follow-up
➤ Encouragement of the patient and informal caregivers related to instructions provided by all disciplines involved

The physician can improve the quality of the home care team and strengthen teamwork by volunteering to serve on the agency's clinical review committee, quality improvement committee, or other committees affecting clinical care. The physician can also improve quality by giving lectures at agency in-service educational programs for nurses and other professional staff. Finally, always remember that the most important members of the home care team are the patient, family and caregivers. Professional team members should make every effort to support them.

PRIVACY AND CONFIDENTIALITY ISSUES

The Health Insurance Portability and Accountability Act (HIPAA) does not require formal or written patient consent for physicians to communicate with home health providers for the purpose of coordination and ongoing care. All communications with HHAs are confidential. Patient-related documents received from the HHA should be filed in the medical record. Use of the Internet to communicate with HHAs and caregivers must be conducted on HIPAA-compliant systems or must be with the consent of the patient.

RESOURCES

Medicare Benefit and Policy Manual Chapter 7-Home Health Services. www.cms.gov/manuals/ Downloads/bp102c07.pdf

CMS Medicare and Home Health Care: http://www.medicare.gov/publications/pubs/pdf/10969.pdf

American Academy of Home Care Physicians' *Making Home Care Work in a Medical Practice: A Brief Guide to Reimbursement and Regulations* (Revised January 2011, www.aahcp.org)

CHAPTER | SIX

Choosing and Evaluating Organizations that Provide Services in the Home

After reading this chapter you should be able to:

1. Summarize the steps for selecting a Medicare-certified home health agency

2. Recognize services that may be provided by home health agencies

3. Identify additional types of home care, private duty, and ancillary services that may be available to help home care patients

4. Describe the process of selecting a durable medical equipment supplier

Many services can aid home care patients, their families and their caregivers. These include but are not limited to home health agencies (HHAs), social service agencies, private duty services, and durable medical equipment (DME) companies. This chapter describes how to obtain quality services for home care patients.

SELECTING A MEDICARE-CERTIFIED HOME HEALTH AGENCY

When selecting an HHA, physicians should exercise the same care they use to select the hospitals with which they are affiliated. Physicians often need to use several agencies to ensure geographic coverage and appropriate services for all their patients. In most regions, there are several agencies providing similar services; the challenge for the referring physician is how to select the best providers. The referring physician is responsible for selecting an organization that provides high-quality care that meets all of the patient's skilled home care needs. On-site visits to an HHA may help in assessing its capability and in providing the opportunity to ask key questions (see Table 1; these questions can also be sent and answered by mail or email). A prudent due diligence process will help a referring physician choose among the many HHAs available. The proper HHA will provide the best quality health care that is effective, efficient, safe and timely. This will translate to measurable outcomes that will prevent frequent emergency room visits and hospitalizations.

TABLE 1 Key questions to ask a home health agency

- ➤ What are the agency's accreditations? Accreditation, a voluntary process, signifies that an agency meets national standards. Organizations offering such certification include The Joint Commission (www.jointcommission.org) and the Community Health Accreditation Program (CHAP; www.chapinc.org).

- ➤ What are the results of state and federal surveys? This information can be found at Home Health Compare, a quality initiative of the Centers for Medicare & Medicaid Services (CMS) that compares HHA outcomes (www.medicare.gov/homehealthcompare).

- ➤ What is the range of services? Does the agency have a wide range of providers on staff, or does it use subcontractors? How does the agency communicate with and manage subcontractors? What are the nurse-to-patient and therapist-to-patient ratios? Does the agency have a particular niche or specialization that more appropriately meets the needs of select patients or diagnoses?

- ➤ How long has the agency been in business and what is its general reputation in the community?

- ➤ Are there appropriate policies, procedures, and care management protocols?

- ➤ What type of medical insurance does the agency accept (Medicare, Medicaid, managed care, workman's compensation, private insurance, private pay)? What are the agency's policies for coverage of underinsured or uninsured patients?

- ➤ What is the referral process? What is the agency's general response time?

- ➤ How is the agency managed? Who are its directors, director of nursing, medical director, and other key personnel?

- ➤ How are weekend and "after business hours" communications between nurses and physicians handled? During evening and weekend management of complex cases, it is preferable to choose an HHA that allows telephone access to the patient's primary nurse rather than only to an "on-call" nurse.

➤ When patients are sick on the weekend, what type of staff is available to visit the home? This question reflects the agency's ability to decrease the need for home-bound patients to make weekend visits to the emergency department. Regarding opening new cases, HHA personnel should be able to visit a new patient on any weekend of the year.

➤ How does the agency coordinate care among its field staff (e.g., nurses, physical therapists, occupational therapists) and the referring physician?

➤ The old model of HHAs provides little in the way of involving physicians in home care. Superior models now include various interfaces with the referring physician, especially if he or she is performing house calls.

➤ What is the agency's capacity and experience in dealing with special populations (e.g., pediatrics, individuals with HIV/AIDS)?

Numerous quality factors can assist the physician in choosing the right HHA. Centers for Medicare & Medicaid Services (CMS) has instituted quality health care initiatives that identify the outcomes of patient care provided by certified HHAs based on publicly reported data. These data come from Medicare's Outcome and Assessment Information Set (OASIS-C) taken upon admission and discharge from the HHA. Eleven OASIS-C outcomes are publicly reported on www.medicare.gov/homehealthcompare, i.e., acute care hospitalization, ambulation/locomotion, emergent care, bathing, discharge to community, dyspnea, oral medications, pain interfering with activity, status of wounds, transferring and urinary incontinence. An HHA quality checklist based on the questions in Table 1 can be used. Table 2 lists resources for finding HHAs.

As a practical consideration, some agencies may have serious limitations in regard to the availability of their physical, occupational, and speech therapists. Before referral, the physician should ascertain whether a therapist is available, the level of training and expertise, how long a delay is anticipated before services can start, and at what frequency per week the agency can provide therapy staff.

TABLE 2 Finding a home health agency

➤ www.medicare.gov/homehealthcompare: Uses a zip code to identify all Medicare-certified agencies in an area.

➤ State Departments on Aging (see Chapter 17)

➤ Local Area Agencies on Aging/social services

➤ Hospital discharge planners

➤ National Association for Home Care & Hospice (NAHC) (www.nahc.org)

➤ Patient's choice of HHA

TABLE 3 Health care professionals who may provide their services through a home health agency

> ➤ Registered nurse (RN), medical or surgical

> ➤ Certified WOCN nurse (wound/ostomy/continence nurse; previously known as an enterostomal nurse (ET) nurse)

> ➤ Certified infusion nurse

> ➤ Certified psychiatric nurse

> ➤ Certified diabetic educator (either nurse or dietitian)

> ➤ Physical therapist

> ➤ Occupational therapist

> ➤ Medical social worker

> ➤ Registered dietitian

> ➤ Speech therapist

> ➤ Home health aide

> ➤ Licensed practical nurse (LPN) or licensed vocational nurse (LVN) (under supervision of a registered nurse)

> ➤ Physical therapy assistant (under supervision of a physical therapist)

If the proposed service cannot meet the patient's needs, the physician must try to find another HHA that can provide the appropriate skill level, frequency and duration of services. Table 3 lists services that may be provided by an HHA.

The physician often plays a more passive role in selecting an HHA for follow-up after a hospitalization. While physician input is critical in determining the scope of home care, hospitalized patients usually have a discharge planner assisting them in choosing an HHA. Medicare-participating hospitals, as part of their discharge planning evaluations, are required to provide Medicare beneficiaries with a list of Medicare-certified HHAs or organizations that serve the patient's geographic area.

OTHER HOME SERVICES

The same care and attention to quality should be part of the process in selecting organizations to provide services, such as:

➤ Laboratory/x-ray and other ancillary services

➤ Pharmacy

➤ Private-duty nursing services

➤ Homemaker services

➤ Specialized high-technology services

Many of these providers are not Medicare-certified, but some have state licenses or are accredited by entities such as The Joint Commission, the Community Health Accreditation Program (CHAP), or the Clinical Laboratory Improvement Amendments (CLIA). These organizations should keep records on each patient they serve that are more extensive than the forms they send to the physician for signature. A physician who wishes to learn more about the quality of these organizations can ask to see the record resulting from his or her referral.

Private-duty nursing and homemaker services are particularly unregulated and referring physicians need to be especially prudent in evaluating these services prior to recommending them to a patient (Table 4).

There has been a dramatic increase in the number of assisted living facilities (ALFs) over the past two decades. As of January 1, 2006, Medicare payments for physician visits to ALFs doubled because of higher level evaluation and management (E/M) codes and increased payments. This has resulted in a dramatic rise of physician visits to ALFs. See Table 5 for questions to ask before referring home care patients to ALFs or agreeing to see patients in these facilities.

TABLE 4 Questions for the private-duty agency

➤ What are the rates for services? Charges for care should be quoted on an hourly, daily, or live-in basis.

➤ What hours can be arranged? Determine daily minimum and maximum hours available and flexibility in arranging split shifts. For example, some patients may require two shifts of three hours, for a total of six hours a day. Other patients may require continuous staffing 24 hours a day, seven days a week.

➤ Is staff bonded and insured? Patients or families should be encouraged to ask the agency to provide documentation.

➤ If the patient or family is dissatisfied with the staff, are substitutes available?

TABLE 5 Questions to ask assisted living facilities

➤ What hours are staffed by nurses?

➤ What services are nurses able to provide (some state regulations and ALF policies restrict nurses from, for example, performing wound care or administering enemas or suppositories)?

(Continued)

TABLE 5 *Continued*

➤ Can the AFL provide special diets?

➤ What other services are available onsite? This can include phlebotomy (very helpful), physical, occupational and speech therapy, psychiatry, podiatry, audiology, optometry, etc.

➤ Does the AFL have a special dementia unit? A secured (locked) unit?

➤ What level of functionally impaired patient will the AFL take? Wheel chair bound? Foley catheter? G-tube fed patient?

➤ For what reasons does the ALF insist on discharging residents? Will the ALF allow residents to enroll in hospice and die on-site?

TABLE 6 Questions to determine the quality of durable medical equipment providers

➤ Which DME organizations have provided the highest quality service? Does the DME provider have a reputation of adequately teaching the patient and family how to utilize equipment that is delivered to the home? Can the DME provider quickly deliver urgently needed products such as oxygen and wound care supplies?

➤ What is the range of services provided by the DME provider?

➤ How does the DME provider deal with equipment maintenance? Are repair costs included? Does it loan equipment during repairs?

➤ How is paperwork handled (e.g Certificates of Medical Necessity (CMNs))?

➤ How does the DME supplier collaborate with HHAs and hospices?

DURABLE MEDICAL EQUIPMENT

When utilizing organizations that provide durable medical equipment (DME), an efficient way to perform due diligence is to question the nursing administrators of several local HHAs. Larger agencies may have a greater ability to provide the physician with recommendations of several reliable DME providers.

CONCLUSION

Quality home health care is a top priority. Its goal is to improve patients' functional and physical outcomes so they can achieve and maintain independence in their home environment. Choosing the right HHA and other ancillary services can make a significant impact in improving the quality of life for these patients.

RESOURCES

Centers for Medicare & Medicaid Services (www.cms.gov)

Home Health Compare (www.medicare.gov/homehealthcompare)

American Association of Home Care (www.aahomecare.org)

The Joint Commission (www.jointcommission.org)

Community Health Accreditation Program (CHAP) (www.chapinc.org)

National Association for Home Care & Hospice (NAHC) (www.nahc.org)

American Association of Home Care (DME information) (www.aahomecare.org)

American Academy of Home Care Physicians (www.aahcp.org)

CHAPTER SEVEN

Case Management: Making Use of Community Resources

After reading this chapter you should be able to:

1. Define case management and identify who can function in the role of case manager

2. Describe how to find available community resources to aid in case management

An important goal of health care is fostering patient independence in self-care (i.e., the patient manages his or her own care). A remarkable array of goods and services are available for the home care patient, which can make the task of coordinating them challenging. When the patient's health problems worsen and he or she becomes dependent on others, assistance with management and decision-making may be necessary. Case management includes those activities necessary to determine the patient's needs, arrange for and coordinate the appropriate services, and monitor the effectiveness of services and reassess them as needed.[1] In addition to the physician, case managers can come from a nursing, social work, or fiduciary background. Case management may focus on supportive services (to meet daily living needs) or health care services that can be general or oriented to particular diseases (i.e., disease management). Disease management generally involves specially trained nurse case managers to implement detailed clinical protocols in managing specific chronic medical conditions.[2]

Effective case management focuses on integrating care across subspecialty and medical-social boundaries. Home care-based case management programs can have a significant impact on hospitalization and costs.[3,4] Likewise, some specialized disease management programs have been shown to be cost-effective

TABLE 1 The levels of case management

➤ The patient is his or her own case manager.

➤ The patient needs assistance from family members or significant others in planning/coordinating care.

➤ Problems are too complex for the family to deal with alone, but can be managed with regular input from the treating physician.

➤ For the most complex levels of care, a multidisciplinary professional team is needed to assist the patient and family. Such a team should have a designated case manager/team leader.

➤ Flexibility is needed to move between levels of case management with the ultimate goal of patient independence and continuity of care.

for selected populations (e.g., heart failure patients).[5] These findings are not universal, however. One study failed to demonstrate reduced use or cost of health care for high-risk older people, but noted that other potentially favorable effects of this type of case management need to be evaluated.[6] It is important, therefore, to assess the individual patient's needs carefully and understand the limits and abilities of specific case or disease management programs.

A particularly critical time for case management services is when a homebound patient transitions from being in the hospital to returning home. In an effort to improve care transitions, many hospitals are identifying at-risk patients early and implementing care management programs to prevent adverse events after hospital discharge. The Enhanced Discharge Planning Program (EDPP) of Rush University Medical Center's Older Adult Programs is an example of such a program. EDPP provides short-term telephonic care coordination from a master's level social worker within 72 hours of discharge. The social worker assesses the post-discharge situation and intervenes to ensure the discharge plan of care is happening as planned and links patients to long-term supports in their community. More information is available at http://www.hpoe.org/case-studies/4340001768.

Homebound patients often have both medical and supportive care needs that must be addressed. Services can be accessed through the health side (e.g., the physician office or home health agency) or through the supportive services side (e.g., through the local Area Agency on Aging (AAA) or private geriatric case managers). Services through the local AAA can include Meals on Wheels, homemaker services, home modification, prescription assistance, utility assistance, elder abuse services and others. During the past five years, a significant expansion in home and community services has occurred in most states. Many states now offer relatively high-technology support (e.g., components of "smart homes") to assist elders to remain in the community. The goal of these services is not only to improve care and enable community dwelling, but also to reduce the propensity toward institutionalization.

In recent years there has been a significant shift in the provision of home and community-based care from agency-delivered services to consumers directing their own care—with administrative assistance from the AAA or a fiscal intermediary.[7,8] In consumer-directed care, consumers are the employers of their assistants and direct their own care plan with some oversight by the AAA. As consumer-directed care expands, it is important that physicians assess their patients' capacity to make decisions to direct their own care.

Physicians are a crucial link to community resources, and the physician with a well-trained office staff may serve many of the roles of a case manager. Patients traditionally rely on their physician to inform, order, supervise, and coordinate the many services that are instrumental to successful home care programs. Furthermore, the health care system is structured to require a patient's physician to order needed services. Many patients and families turn to their physician for advice when they perceive the need for additional resources. Seventy-eight percent of patients requiring care in their home receive all their needed assistance from family and friends.[9] The physician may be the only health professional who provides care and advice in these cases. He or she can function effectively in this role for most patients with a resultant decrease in costs and increase in quality.[10]

In more complicated cases, the physician may encourage the use of a designated case manager. Patients with problem behaviors, greater functional disability, informal support problems, and problems with service provider agencies have been shown to require a higher level of case management.[11] A variety of agencies—governmental, not-for-profit, and for profit—offer case management services; consequently, it is important for physicians to become familiar with these resources in the community. Information on geriatric care managers can be found at the National Association of Professional Geriatric Care Managers at www.caremanager.org.

Recognition of the frequent interdependence of supportive living services and complex health care management has led to a number of programs designed to bridge walls between the two. These include some links between state waiver programs and special needs plans (operated under Medicare Part C), and the Program for All-Inclusive Care of the Elderly (PACE). A number of AAAs are developing links with local medical groups to enhance integration.[12,13]

COMMUNITY RESOURCES

State and local information and referral services provide the physician and patient or caregiver with access to national and local disease-specific charitable organizations and advocacy groups that can provide additional resources. A useful first step in sorting through the variety of goods and services available for a home care patient is the U.S. Department of Health and Human Services' Administration on Aging web site (www.aoa.gov). Under the direction of the

Administration on Aging, there are state units for each state and territory, as well as AAAs. Chapter 17 lists the State Departments on Aging with their contact information.

The Eldercare Locator at (800) 677-1116 or www.eldercare.gov, is an information and referral service that enables callers to access the names and locations of AAAs and other entities that may be able to provide resource information. For patients under age 60 years, the state departments of human resources, health, social services, or vocational rehabilitation may be contacted. Although the federal or state funding sources differ for different age groups, the local providers of services are often the same.

For children with special needs, there are additional resources, such as:

➤ Early intervention programs

➤ Rehabilitation with multiple therapies

➤ School-based educational/developmental programs [14]

Information about these programs can be obtained through local and state agencies established through the Association of Maternal and Child Health Programs (www.amchp.org). To locate an agency in a particular area, call (202) 775-0436.

Considerable local variation in availability exists, but most programs will have information and referral services and some or all of the services listed in Table 2.

TABLE 2 Access, community-based, and other services

Access services
➤ Information and referral
➤ Transportation
➤ Outreach services
➤ Case management
➤ Escort services
➤ Electronic databases for pharmacy, etc.
Community-based services
➤ Day care
➤ Elder abuse protective services
➤ Senior centers
➤ Respite services

➤ Congregate nutrition programs

➤ Legal assistance

➤ Congregate housing

Services to residents of nursing homes and other care-providing facilities

➤ Long-term care ombudsman program

➤ Support for elderly persons with Alzheimer's disease and their families

➤ Housing services

➤ Employment services

➤ Health/fitness programs

➤ Rehabilitation services, including vocational rehabilitation and special education

➤ Energy assistance

➤ Counseling

➤ Senior companions

➤ Foster grandparents, foster homes

➤ Volunteer programs

➤ Self-help/support groups

➤ Housing services

➤ Crime prevention/victim assistance

In-home services

➤ Home health services

➤ Skilled nursing

➤ Physical and occupational therapy

➤ Speech therapy

➤ Medical social services

➤ Nutritional guidance

➤ Home health aide

➤ Telephone reassurance

➤ Hospice services

➤ Homemaker/personal care services

(Continued)

TABLE 2 *Continued*

➤ Chores/housekeeping

➤ Home repair

➤ Home delivered meals/Meals on Wheels

➤ Medical equipment and supplies

➤ Friendly visitor

➤ Portable electronic devices for communication and monitoring

Diagnostic services

➤ Portable x-ray

➤ Mobile ultrasound

➤ Portable laboratory instruments and mobile laboratories

➤ Home blood-drawing services

➤ Telemonitoring services networked through congregate housing structures

➤ Sleep study

REFERENCES

1. Fanale SE, Hepburn KW, Sternberg TV. Care management. *J Am Geriatr Soc.* 1991;34: 431–437.

2. DeBusk RF, West JA, Miller NH, Taylor CB. Chronic disease management: treating the patient with disease(s) vs. treating disease(s) in the patient. *Arch Intern Med.* 1999;159:2739–2742.

3. Landi F, Gambassi G, Pola R, Tabaccanti S, Cavinato T, Carbonin PU, Bernabei R. Impact of integrated home care services on hospital use. *J Am Geriatr Soc.* 1999;47:1430–1434.

4. Duke C. The frail elderly community-based case management project. *Geriatric Nursing.* 2005;26(2):122–127.

5. Ahmed A. Quality and outcomes of heart failure care in older adults: role of multidisciplinary disease-management programs. *J Am Geriatr Soc.* 2002;50:1590–1593.

6. Boult C, Rassen J, Rassen A, Moore RJ, Robison S. The effect of case management on the costs of health care for enrollees in Medicare Plus Choice plans: a randomized trial. *J Am Geriatr Soc.* 2000;48:996–1001.

7. Bengamin A.E. Consumer-directed services at home: A new model for persons with disabilities. *Health Affairs.* 2001:20(6);80–95.

8. Doty P. *Consumer-Directed Home Care: Effects on Family Caregivers.* San Francisco, CA: National Center on Caregiving Family Caregiver Alliance. 2004.

9. Thompson L. *Long-term care: support for family caregivers.* Washington, DC: Georgetown University Long-Term Care Financing Project. March 2004.

10. Goldberg AI, Trubitt MJ. An integrated approach to home health care. *Physician Executive.* 1994;25:45–46.

11. Diwan S. Allocation of case management resources in long-term care: predicting high use of case management time. *Gerontologist.* 1999;39:580–590.

12. Kinosian B, Yudin J, Danish A, Touzel S. Elder partnership for all inclusive care (Elder-PAC): 5 year follow-up of integrating care for frail, community elders, linking home based primary care with an Area Agency on Aging (AAA) as an independence at home model. *J Am Geriatr Soc.* 2010,Volume 58, Issue Supplement s1, 56. Article first published online: 1 APR 2010.

13. Counsell SR, Callahan CM, Clark DO, Tu W, Buttar AB, Stump TE, Ricketts GD. Bariatric case management for low income seniors: A randomized controlled trial. *JAMA.* 2007;298(22):2623–2630.

14. Johnson CP, Blasco PA. Community resources for children with special health care needs. *Pediatr Ann.* 1997;26:679–686.

CHAPTER | EIGHT

Care Transitions

After reading this chapter you should be able to:

1. Define the term "care transition" and summarize its importance in the fragmented health care system

2. Recognize the processes needed to create successful care transitions

3. Identify the variety of health care professionals involved in care transitions

4. Explain how quality care transitions can reduce hospital readmissions

The inherent fragmentation of 21st century medicine has moved care transitions to the forefront of the health care agenda. Well-crafted definitions of the term "care transitions" currently exist including the National Transitions of Care Coalition definition: "care involved when a patient/client leaves one care setting (i.e., hospital, nursing home, assisted living facility, SNF [skilled nursing facility], primary care physician, home health, or specialist) and moves to another"[1]; and the American Geriatrics Society definition: "a set of actions designed to ensure the coordination of care as patients transfer between different locations."[2]

More important is the realization that a transition of care occurs with every change in site of care (even within the same institution as from surgery to postoperative ward) or caregiver (primary care to specialist, nursing shift changes, and so forth) and thus demands a thoughtful handoff from the current to the next provider. For example, in a hospital discharge this includes not just the physical move from hospital to home, but from attending hospital physician to community physician, hospital nurses to home health nurses, hospital physical therapists to home health physical therapist, hospital pharmacist to community pharmacist, and all other counterparts within the health care delivery system. How all of these entities communicate in order to provide timely and appropriate transfer of pertinent clinical information across licensure and roles is paramount for success. Availability of all involved providers for discussion before and after the transition occurs will determine the degree of success of the transition.

The emergence of care transitions is related to both quality and finances. Thirty-nine million community hospital discharges occur annually according to 2006 national statistics on outcomes for all discharges from the Agency for Healthcare Research and Quality Healthcare Cost and Utilization Project.[3] Some 9.91% of hospital discharge patients receive home health care (AHRQ HCUPnet, 2009 [on-line]). The quality and financial concerns with these hospital discharge care transitions are secondary to the high rate of readmissions. Medicare claims data from 2003–2004 regarding hospital discharges indicate that 19.6% of those discharged were readmitted within 30 days and 34% were readmitted within 60 days; 90% of readmissions were estimated to be unplanned. While the "correct" readmission rate is unknown, the current high return rate cost to Medicare for unplanned readmissions was $17.4 billion in 2004.[4] These statistics have prompted the Centers for Medicare & Medicaid Services (CMS) to implement actions that will penalize high readmission rates, encourage improved transitions of care and increasingly impact the home care practice.

CREATING A SUCCESSFUL TRANSITION

Determining what constitutes a successful outcome in any individual transition is difficult. For one patient, contentment is a peaceful death; for another, the desired outcome is a return to full time employment; and for a third, happiness is the ability to resume care for a treasured pet. The transition must be tailored to the patient/family need rather than the patient being "shoehorned" into the existing discharge process. Until outcome measures are available to guide best practices, care transitions should follow consensus recommendations by groups such as the National Transitions of Care Coalition and the American Medical Directors Association (AMDA) Clinical Practice Guidelines for Transitions of Care through the Long-Term Care Continuum.

TABLE 1 Elements that should be part of every home transition

The site sending the patient maintains responsibility and/or availability for the patient until the receiving site assumes care
Patient-centered focus
➤ Patient/family participates in decisions
➤ Critical information arrives with or prior to the patient
➤ Clinical information moves with the patient

Medication reconciliation

➤ Performed by sending and receiving entities at every transition

➤ Involves every drug taken: prescription, nonprescription, over-the-counter, herbals, vitamins and those belonging to others

Establish advance directives

➤ Seek answers on deeper issues than resuscitation: whether return to the hospital is desired, whether antibiotics are to be given, whether tube feeding should ever be instituted and other end-of-life treatment wishes. These decisions can be established and documented through a variety of documents, which include:

> ➤ The advance directive document Five Wishes®, a legal power of attorney for health care accepted in 40 states guides patients/families through many of these issues;

> ➤ The POLST (Physician Orders for Life Sustaining Treatment) form-legally accepted as a physician order in eight states and being considered in more than 20 other states; or

> ➤ The DNAR/DNR (Do Not Attempt Resuscitation/Do Not Resuscitate) form

Communication

➤ Timely, crucial information must be shared between clinicians from the sending team to the receiving team, and between team members at both sending and receiving sites.

➤ Clinician-to-clinician conversations are the gold standard of communication, and the effectiveness of care coordination is determined by the quality, not the quantity, of these interactions.

➤ Patients and their families assume clinicians are sharing critical information on their care; they should not be disappointed

Interdisciplinary in nature

➤ Everyone involved in the transition, regardless of licensure and position, is involved, accountable and responsive.

Patient safety/environmental issues in the home. Examples include:

➤ Safety: stairs, fall risk, abusive domestic individuals, sensory impairments

➤ Support: Is it available, who provides it, is the patient a caregiver for others?

➤ Finances: can the patient afford medications, providers, food and medical supplies?

➤ Transportation: how will the patient pick up medications and food and get to medical appointments?

NEW FACES IN THE TRANSITION PROCESS

Heightened awareness of transitioning patients means the community physician will interact with a new array of health care system licensures and positions. Case management, performed by those known as case managers, discharge planners, care managers, social workers or others, is moving beyond the old "discharge planning" paradigm to active engagement in post-hospital activity. The physician should expect to be contacted by these individuals as they schedule physician appointments, perform medication reconciliation, ensure laboratory and radiology follow-up and arrange specialty referrals for patients leaving the hospital.

An expanding role of pharmacists will continue both in review of hospital patient medications as patients leave the institution, and in follow up with post-hospital/ skilled nursing facility admissions. This is especially important because of the findings that older patients regularly have medication discrepancies upon leaving the hospital[5] and that such discrepancies more than double the likelihood of rehospitalization within 30-days.[6] There is also mounting evidence that pharmacy involvement in transitioning patient medication alignment can reduce preventable adverse drug events, emergency department visits, hospital readmissions and mortality.[7]

As new care transition programs spring up across the country, many employ nurses – typically advance practice nurses – to follow patients across sites of care. Programs based on the work of Dr. Eric Coleman Care Transitions Program (www.caretransitions.org) and Dr. Mary Naylor Transitional Care Model (www.transitionalcare.info), as well as the programs of "Guided Care" at Johns Hopkins in Baltimore (www.guidedcare.org), "Heart Care At Home" through the Cleveland Clinic, and many more are employing nurse clinicians to maintain contact with participants. These nurses act as information sources for new clinicians, coach patients and families on how to best interact with clinicians, monitor medications and facilitate communication between the multiple practitioners involved in an individual patient's care.

Hospitals are aggressively addressing hospital returns in response to looming financial penalties for 30-day readmissions. In the Re-Engineered Discharge (RED) (www.bu.edu/fammed/projectred/) program at Boston University Medical Center patient education before leaving the hospital is coupled with instructions on next steps in care, and an expedited Transition Summary. The Transition Summary is a "quick and dirty" summary of why the patient was in the hospital, and provides critical information for immediate use in patient care, including medications and next steps. It should accompany the patient to the next site of care. Similarly, Project BOOST (Better Outcomes for Older Adults through Safe Transitions - www.hospitalmedicine.org), created by the Society for Hospital Medicine to reduce 30-day readmissions through patient/family education and preparedness, medication reconciliation, communicating with community providers and post-hospital telephone contacts anticipates safer transfers home from the hospital. The physician will increasingly encounter programs such as these.

The most important component of successful care transitions is the oldest; that of an educated empowered patient and family. The patient-centered model of care is focused on the patient/family maintaining their own medication list and medical history, then using that information in a positive fashion to assist the clinical team to create a care plan that reflects the patient's needs and belief system. The difficulty for the community physician is to mesh these component parts into a care team that works together for the patient instead of disparately.

New interactions inevitably require dealing with new forms. No regional or national standards for a care transfer form exist. Additionally, the quality and quantity of information received will vary widely. Proactively engaging local hospitals with feedback on current forms and suggestions for improvements offers the opportunity to modify the process to the benefit of the community physician and patients.

HOSPITAL READMISSIONS AND HOUSE CALLS

No area is currently under more intense scrutiny, especially from CMS, than readmission to the hospital within 30 days of discharge. The home care physician will enhance his or her value significantly, and become a provider of first choice, by avoiding unnecessary hospital readmissions.

The Patient Protection and Affordable Care Act (PPACA), signed March 23, 2010, promises to substantially change home care practices. Section 3001/3006 indicates that the U.S. Health and Human Services Secretary will "develop a plan" for incentives and efficiency measures for home health care, and the act requires

TABLE 2 Generally accepted methods to reduce unwarranted hospital readmissions

➤ Recognize the patient's need for continuing medical, nursing and supportive care after discharge, arrange for appropriate services

➤ Determine and respect advance directives

➤ Maintain clear communication with the patient/family and the home health agency (HHA) on best methods to contact the physician, and respond in a timely fashion

➤ Work with the HHA on physician notification. Accepted tools that may be modified minimally or directly used for home care include the Interact II and the AMDA Acute Change of Condition in the Long-Term Care Setting guideline (see Resources at the end of this chapter).

use of an electronic health record by 2014. Further possible changes relating to care transitions are found throughout the law. The rules and regulations that will enforce these provisions and the indicators that will measure how well home health care is applied by providers are yet to be written.

Opportunities for home care involvement in care transitions exist within the PPACA as well. CMS will increasingly move to payment based on good outcomes, or value-based purchasing, rather than by volume. Hospitals with excess preventable readmissions within 30 days of discharge will begin to receive reduced reimbursements beginning in 2012, and declines in reimbursement to poorly performing physicians will likewise follow. Additionally, in 2015, hospitals will receive 1% lower payments if patients develop avoidable hospital-acquired conditions. Physicians with house call practices that perform well will receive augmented reimbursement by Medicare and may anticipate higher patient volume resulting from becoming a sought-after provider. There may be opportunities to partner with hospitals to share in savings through Accountable Care Organizations (ACOs) and other models. Another provision in the PPACA that could impact home care is the Community-based Care Transitions Program (CCTP). The CCTP, mandated by section 3026, provides funding to test models for improving care transitions for high-risk Medicare beneficiaries. The goals of the CCTP are to improve transitions of beneficiaries from the inpatient hospital setting to other care settings, to improve quality of care, to reduce readmissions for high risk beneficiaries, and to document measureable savings to the Medicare program. The CCTP is part of Partnership for Patients, a national patient safety initiative through which the Administration is supporting broad-based efforts to reduce harm caused to patients in hospitals and improve care transitions (www .cms.gov/demoprojectsevalrpts/md/itemdetail.asp?itemid=CMS1239313).

There are other initiatives such as the Independence at Home Demonstration Program (PPACA Section 3024), which provides shared cost savings between Medicare and house call programs for patients with multiple, chronic conditions to receive coordinated primary care services in lower cost settings such as the home. Carving out a role for house call practices into newer concepts such as Independence at Home (IAH), Accountable Care Organizations (ACO) or a Patient-Centered Medical Home (PCMH) model will open doors for both physicians and their patients to achieve better outcomes of care.

The resurgence of a well-regarded family of programs, the patient-centered medical home (PCMH), also holds promise. PCMH programs involve a physician-led team of health professionals that either provides or coordinates all aspects of the patient's preventive, acute and chronic care needs across settings and practitioners. PCMHs seek to integrate patients and families as active participants in their own health and well-being by developing sustained partnerships with them. PCMHs strive to achieve the following:

➤ Serve as an accessible first contact care or entry point to the health care system for the majority of a person's health care needs.

➤ Maintain a continuous relationship with the patient over time.

➤ Provide comprehensive care that meets or arranges for most of a patient's health care needs.

➤ Coordinate care across a patient's conditions, providers and settings in consultation with the patient and caregivers/family members.

As such, the PCMH potentially has the ability to enhance the outcome of the episode of care over multiple care settings for the patient and caregivers.

RESOURCES

National Transitions of Care Coalition (NTOCC) (www.ntocc.org)

Transitions of Care in the Long-Term Care Continuum by the American Medical Directors Association (AMDA) (www.amda.com/tools/clinical/transitionsofcare.cfm)

American Academy of Home Care Physicians (AAHCP) (www.aahcp.org)

West Virginia Home Health Quality Initiative (www.homehealthquality.org)

Interact II: Working Together to Improve Care and Reduce Acute Care Transfers (www.interact .geriu.org)

American Medical Directors Association (AMDA) Acute Change of Condition in the Long-Term Care Setting guideline – available through www.amda.com

Medical home and self assessment tools

  www.medicalhomeinfo.org

  www.medicalhomeimprovement.org

  www.ncqa.org/tabid/631/default.aspx

REFERENCES

1. National Transitions of Care Coalition web site. http://www.ntocc.org. Accessed September 21, 2011.

2. Coleman EA, Boult C. Improving the quality of transitional care for persons with complex care needs. Position statement of the American Geriatrics Society health care systems committee. *J Am Geriatr Soc.* 2003;51(4):556–557.

3. Agency for Healthcare Research and Quality Statistics on Hospital Stays web site. Agency for Healthcare Research and Quality Healthcare Cost and Utilization Project. http://www .hcupnet.ahrq.gov. Accessed September 21, 2011.

4. Jencks S, Williams M, Coleman E. Re-hospitalizations among patients in the Medicare fee-for-service program. *N Engl J Med.* 2009;360:1418–28.

5. Bell CM, Brener SS, Gunraj N, Huo C, Bierman AS, Scales DC, Bajcar J, Zwarenstein M, Urbach DR. Association of ICU or hospital admission with unintentional discontinuation of medications for chronic diseases. *JAMA.* 2011:306(8):840–847.

6. Coleman EA, Smith JD, Devbani R, Sung-joon M; Posthospital medication discrepancies: Prevalence and contributing factors. *Arch Intern Med.* 2005;165:1842–1847.

7. Schnipper JL, Kirwin JL, Cotugno MC, Wahlstrom SA, et al. Role of pharmacist counseling in preventing adverse drug events after hospitalization. *Arch Intern Med.* 2006;166:565–571.

CHAPTER | NINE

Special Home Care Populations

After reading this chapter you should be able to:

1. Recognize the wide variety of medical conditions that can be treated at home

2. Discuss the availability of specialized home care services

The need to find the most appropriate and cost-effective ways to manage a wide spectrum of conditions have expanded the repertoire of home care services dramatically. Home care can be a welcome and effective component in the care and management of patients of all ages, from high risk obstetrics, to infants, children, and adults who may have conditions that require the technology, therapies, and/or coordination of care provided by the home care team. The evolving paradigms of payment using global or population-based metrics that rely on high quality, cost-efficient, and patient-centered care will ultimately redirect care from the cost intensive acute and institutional setting to the home or assisted living setting.

This evolution will require physicians to become capable of managing and coordinating care for a variety of conditions, utilizing technology, ancillary health professionals, caregivers, and community resources. The types of patients and conditions that fit into this strategy are diverse and to provide a comprehensive account here would take volumes. The ever-expanding list of the medical, surgical, and psychiatric conditions that can be managed through specialized home care are listed in Table 1. There is significant overlap in disease and care management strategies, and the coordination of care for each of these populations may require a unique mix of medical specialists, home care nursing, and ancillary therapists, as well as specialized medical equipment and community social services and other resources. Unfortunately, one of the most difficult, time consuming, and care-limiting problem is that which pertains to authorization and payment. No matter how effective the care plan, it is futile without adequate resources.

It is important for the physician overseeing the care of these patients to be aware of the capabilities and limitations of available home care providers. Some agencies may have specialized services that facilitate the transition to the home, whereas other problems may not fit into their skill set. The physician may need to bring together a "virtual" team (via e-mail and telephone conference rather than on-site) with representatives from the different programs and professions involved to achieve consensus on a comprehensive plan for some of these complex patients.

Table 2 identifies some of the specialized services provided by home care agencies that should be considered before making a referral.

TABLE 1 Medical categories and specialized home care services

➤ **Cardiology** *Congestive heart failure, deep vein thrombosis, dobutamine infusion, telemetry, electrocardiogram, anticoagulation*

➤ **Critical care (adult and pediatric)** *Home ICU*

➤ **Endocrinology** *Diabetes treatment, education, and monitoring*

➤ **Emergency medicine** *Acute disposition when hospitalization not required or desired*

➤ **Geriatrics** *Complex bio-psychosocial conditions, dementia, developmentally disabled seniors*

➤ **GI** *Parenteral nutrition, enteral feeds, pH probe testing, gastrostomy tube changes*

➤ **Hematology/oncology** *Chemotherapy, pain management, monitoring and treatment of coagulopathies, anemias, hemoglobinopathies, neutropenia*

➤ **Infectious diseases** *Treatment of bacterial, viral, and fungal infections, HIV/AIDS, and other immunodeficiency states*

➤ **Nephrology** *End-stage renal disease, home dialysis, peritoneal dialysis, nutritional assessments and accommodations*

➤ **Neurology** *Stroke, dementia, Alzheimer's, demyelinating diseases such as multiple sclerosis, amyotrophic lateral sclerosis, Guillian-Barré; physical therapy, occupational therapy, speech and oral motor therapy*

➤ **Obstetrics** *High-risk pregnancy, fetal monitoring, post-partum care, lactation assistance, counseling and education*

➤ **Ophthalmology** *Pre- and post-operative care; low vision training*

➤ **Otolaryngology** *Pre- and post-operative care*

➤ **Pediatrics** *Neonatal and neonatal intensive care unit services such as apnea monitoring, home mechanical ventilation, oxygen, phototherapy for jaundice, total parenteral nutrition and enteral feeds, developmental assessment and treatment, social services, technology management*

➤ **Pediatric-specific subspecialty** *Care for infectious diseases, pulmonary, neurology, gastroenterology, hematology, oncology, genetics, surgery*

➤ **Podiatry** *Nail and foot care*

➤ **Psychiatry** *Alcohol and substance abuse, depression, mood disorders, psychosis, eating disorders, agoraphobia*

➤ **Pulmonary** *Sleep apnea, sleep studies, continuous positive airway pressure (CPAP), asthma, chronic obstructive pulmonary disease, ventilator management, oxygen*

➤ **Rehabilitation medicine** *Rehabilitation evaluation and management, physical therapy, occupational therapy, speech therapy, recreation therapy, vocational therapy*

➤ **Surgery** *Post-operative management, wound care, enterostomal care, pain management*

➤ **Trauma** *Surgical, rehabilitative, and psychological services*

TABLE 2 Specialized home care services

➤ **Infusion** *IV medications and therapies such as total parenteral nutrition, antibiotics, chemotherapy, and transfusions; catheter placement and maintenance (including PICC (peripherally inserted central catheter) line insertion*

➤ **Palliative care and hospice** *Pain and other symptom management, 24-hour support, volunteer support, bereavement services*

➤ **Pediatric** *Neonatal intensive care- and pediatric intensive care-specialized nursing, developmental services*

➤ **Rehabilitation** *Physical therapy, occupational therapy, speech therapy, orthotics, prosthetics*

➤ **Respiratory** *Tracheostomy care, asthma, ventilator and assisted airway technology*

➤ **Wound care** *Post-operative wounds and drains, stoma care, decubitus ulcers*

GENERAL REFERENCES

Libby RC, Editor. Guidelines for Pediatric Home Health Care, 2nd edition. Elk Grove Village, Illinois: American Academy of Pediatrics; 2009.

Rice R. Home Care Nursing Practice: Concepts and Application, 4th edition. Philadelphia: Mosby, Inc; 2006.

CHAPTER TEN

The Veterans Administration's (VA) Home Based Primary Care (HBPC) Program

After reading this chapter you should be able to:

1. Describe the history, mission and outcomes of the HBPC

2. Differentiate between HBPC and Medicare home health care

3. List other VA services available for home care patients and explain how to enroll in these services

INCEPTION OF HOME BASED PRIMARY CARE (HBPC) IN THE DEPARTMENT OF VETERANS AFFAIRS (VA)

Home Based Primary Care (HBPC) is a unique model of non-institutional care developed in the early 1970's as a pilot project within the Veterans Health Administration (www.va.gov/vhapublications/ViewPublication.asp?pub_ID=1534). Started initially at only a few of the VA's largest medical centers, HBPC has expanded to more than 270 locations across the country. The mission of HBPC is to provide comprehensive, interdisciplinary, primary care in the homes of veterans with serious chronic disease and disability. HBPC targets frail, chronically ill veterans for whom routine clinic-based care is not effective. By providing coordinated care and the integration of diverse services, HBPC assists in improving the quality of life for these vulnerable veterans. HBPC is an important part of the VA's array of services designed to meet the care needs of an ever-increasing number of veterans with complex chronic disease.

The mission is accomplished by the ongoing care and oversight of a physician-supervised interdisciplinary team routinely making contact with the veteran at home. "Home" is defined as "where the veteran resides" and may include an assisted living facility but not a nursing home. Visiting veterans at home allows the team unique insight into each veteran's environment, level of home safety, self care capabilities, and medication management among other factors.

The goal of the HBPC program is to promote each veteran's optimum level of health, independence and safety. HBPC optimizes the veteran's health by supporting both the veteran and the caregiver and by helping them to cope with all aspects of chronic disease. The veteran's quality of life improves through symptom management, social and psychological support, and rehabilitative measures, reducing the need for hospitalization, nursing home care, and both emergency department and outpatient clinic visits. The level of oversight provided by HBPC cannot be accomplished during routine clinic-based care. HBPC provides the needed care and management of these medically complex veterans in harmony with the VA's acute care services, avoiding duplication of services and reducing total health care expenditures.

DIFFERENCES BETWEEN VA HBPC AND STANDARD HOME HEALTH CARE

HBPC differs greatly in target population, processes, and outcomes from home care that is available under federal and state programs such as Medicare and Medicaid. HBPC targets persons with multiple chronic diseases, rather than remedial conditions. The care is comprehensive and longitudinal rather than focused and episodic, and is provided by a physician-supervised interdisciplinary team. While patients must be homebound to receive home health services through Medicare, HBPC does not require veterans to be homebound and encourages them to remain active within their abilities to improve their quality of life. HBPC accepts that patients will decline over time and does not require ongoing improvement for a veteran to remain in the program. While Medicare and Medicaid home health programs have shown no definitive impact on hospital days or total cost, HBPC consistently demonstrates its ability to reduce hospitalizations, emergency department visits and total cost of care.

Any veteran enrolled in VA care is eligible for the HBPC program, provided he or she meets specific clinical criteria (see Table 1). Although some programs may

TABLE 1 Eligibility for VA HBPC

➤ Veterans with complex chronic disease(s) that are not effectively managed in routine clinic-based care and that warrant an interdisciplinary team

➤ Multiple advanced chronic diseases, impaired mobility or cognition

➤ Difficulty keeping clinic appointments because travel is arduous or because of significant mental health conditions

➤ Veterans at high risk of recurrent hospitalization, emergency care and/or nursing home placement

➤ Veterans in need of palliative care for advanced disease states

➤ The veteran and caregiver must be willing to accept HBPC as their primary care provider and coordinator of care

➤ Veteran must live in area serviced by the VA HBPC program and meet safety considerations

have slightly different service areas based on community resources, topography, geography and veteran populations, all HBPC programs remain fundamentally committed to the same mission.

HBPC PROGRAM OPERATION/INTERDISCIPLINARY TEAM

The interdisciplinary team provides the comprehensive care for the HBPC patients at home. Team members include a physician medical director, program director, nurse practitioner or physician assistant, nurse, social worker, rehabilitation therapist, dietitian, pharmacist, and more recently a mental health provider usually a psychologist or psychiatrist. Veterans are seen on average three times per month, with the most frequent visits typically from the nurse, mid-level provider or physician. Other members of the team see the veteran as directed by clinical judgment and the plan of care but no less than annually. The pharmacist assesses the medication list multiple times a year and actively participates in the care planning of the veteran.

Once a veteran is found appropriate for admission to the program, a comprehensive assessment (health history, physical, psychosocial, financial, cultural, spiritual, nutritional, functional, home environment, pain, etc.) is performed by multiple disciplines in the veteran's home. The members of the interdisciplinary team meet at least weekly as a team to discuss specific patients, direct their care, and formulate care plans. The care plan for each veteran includes all problems identified by the team members, the medication profile, and measurable patient-centered objectives for the team to accomplish. The veteran's treatment plan is individualized, based on the veteran's and the caregiver's goals, and is signed by all team members. Participation of the veteran and the caregiver in the development of the treatment plan is essential and each veteran is given a copy of the care plan.

OUTCOMES OF VA HBPC

In 2002 the VA conducted a national analysis of utilization and cost for the veterans who received care in HBPC. This analysis compared the six months prior to enrollment in HBPC with the next six months during HBPC. The results from 11,334 veterans in HBPC included an associated reduction in hospital bed days of care by 62%, and reduction in nursing home bed days of care by 88%. Despite an increase in both HBPC and in VA-paid home health services, the mean total VA cost of care dropped 24%, from $38,000 to $29,000 per patient per year, after accounting for the added costs of HBPC and home health. The VA has since implemented a quality measure for HBPC that continually assesses the impact of HBPC on reducing inpatient utilization comparing VA inpatient utilization during HBPC to the six months prior to enrollment in HBPC. This analysis consistently demonstrates an associated reduction in hospital and nursing home days at every HBPC program. In a recent extensive analysis of combined VA and Medicare utilization, enrollment in VA HBPC was associated with a 24% reduction in VA+Medicare hospital admissions, a 36% reduction in VA+Medicare hospital days, and a 13% reduction in total net VA+Medicare costs of care, after accounting for the costs of HBPC. The greater reduction in hospital days rather than in admissions implies that HBPC is not only effective at reducing the frequency of hospitalizations, but also at shortening the length of hospital stays.

INTEGRATING HBPC AND OTHER VA NON-INSTITUTIONAL PROGRAMS

The VA has a variety of non-institutional programs that may be used as an adjuvant to HBPC. All VA non-institutional long-term care services are available to all enrolled veterans who meet specified clinical criteria and are likely to benefit. Homemaker Home Health Aide (HHHA) is a contracted program in the VA that provides a homemaker or home health aide or a personal aide via a contract with a local home health agency. Homemaker services may include assistance with instrumental activities of daily living (IADLs), such as light housekeeping, meal preparation, grocery shopping, escorting the patient to necessary appointments and ensuring patient safety. Home health aide services may include assistance with activities of daily living (ADLs), such as bathing, toileting, eating, dressing and ambulating or transfers. This type of support may be just enough to allow an elderly couple with limited support to be maintained in their own home.

Respite care services are personal care and supportive services delivered in the home, nursing home, hospital, adult day care center, or assisted living facility, for the express purpose of temporarily relieving the caregiver(s). Respite care services may include various VA-provided services; e.g., HHHA, extended hours in adult day care, or even limited admission to a nursing home.

Care Coordination Home Telehealth (CCHT) is the ongoing monitoring and assessment by VA staff of selected patients using telehealth technologies pro-actively to enable prevention, investigation, and treatment in order to enhance the health of patients and prevent unnecessary and inappropriate utilization of resources. Care coordinators facilitate referrals for appropriate services, such as home health and hospice care, serving as a link between such services and the VA health care system.

Adult Day Health Care (ADHC) is often helpful for veterans with dementia or other disabling conditions by providing a safe environment for several hours a day for the veteran and providing some respite for the caregiver. ADHC is a therapeutically oriented outpatient day program that provides health assessment, rehabilitation and socialization to veterans in a congregate setting. Orders such as for wound care and medication for the veteran may be implemented, and medical information such as vital signs and blood glucose monitored.

Veteran Directed Home and Community-Based Services (VDHCBS) is a program wherein a VA Medical Center purchases a package of consumer-directed services from an entity in the state's aging services network. Through VDHCBS, veterans at risk of nursing home admission decide for themselves what mix of services and goods will best meet their needs to live independently in the community. Veterans are allowed to hire their own aides who may be family members or neighbors.

Skilled home health care can be used to supplement HBPC patients with episodic needs for skilled services, such as daily wound care or administration of intravenous antibiotics, that require intensity of service beyond the capacity of the HBPC team.

Hospice is the final stage of the palliative care continuum in which the primary goal of treatment is comfort rather than cure for patients with advanced disease that is life-limiting and unresponsive to disease-modifying treatment. The VA offers to purchase or provide needed hospice care for all enrolled veterans, in whatever setting is most appropriate.

RESOURCES

Veterans and families who are seeking HBPC or other non-institutional services are encouraged to contact their nearest VA health care facility, and request to speak with a social worker. To find the nearest VA facility, go to: www.va.gov and click on "locations" or go directly to either of the following:

➤ http://www2.va.gov/directory/guide/division_flsh.asp?dnum=1

➤ Home Based Primary Care (HBPC) Program Handbook (1/31/07) www.va.gov/vhapublications/ViewPublication.asp?pub_ID=1534

CHAPTER ELEVEN

Hospice and Palliative Care in the Home

After reading this chapter you should be able to:

1. Describe the philosophy and characteristics of palliative care and hospice

2. Explain the benefits of palliative care and hospice

3. Describe the composition of the hospice team and the physician's responsibilities

4. Explain the Medicare hospice benefit

5. Summarize how to bill when the patient is on hospice

Many home care patients are chronically ill and often are receiving services designed to improve quality of life rather than to prolong life. They are especially likely to need palliative care and/or hospice. While many use these terms interchangeably, they are really facets of the same philosophy of medicine expressed so eloquently by Hippocrates, "to cure sometimes, to care often, to comfort always." Palliative care may be given with or without the use of hospice and refers to care designed to relieve distressing symptoms, rather than with a curative goal as its primary objective. It is not merely for the terminally ill, but for everyone who is suffering at any stage of life.

Hospice is a philosophy of care that provides palliation of symptoms at the end of life. Its goal is to help the dying person and his or family and loved ones find meaning in their existence, ending life's journey with dignity and in comfort. Hospice includes physical, psychological, social and spiritual care for dying patients and their families. Hospice strives to allow the person to die in their own home if that is the patient's wish. It may include common palliative measures or more aggressive palliative services such as radiation therapy, surgery or hospitalization for other medical problems (e.g., fixation of a painful fracture). While many believe hospice is mainly for cancer patients, it is also appropriate for

TABLE 1 Characteristics of hospice care

➤ Goal is for comfort care (palliative rather than curative)

➤ Coordination is by an interdisciplinary team (medical director, nurse, care aide, social worker, therapists, spiritual advisor, volunteer)

➤ Support is provided for the family

➤ Pain and other symptoms are controlled

➤ Family counseling and bereavement services are available for one year after the patient's death

➤ The patient must elect the hospice benefit for the terminal illness instead of the standard Medicare benefit

➤ The patient's life expectancy is six months or less if his or her disease follows its natural course

other end-stage conditions such as chronic obstructive pulmonary disease, heart failure, dementia, or any other condition that is in a terminal phase. Hospice is also an insurance benefit and may be a physical building, as in an inpatient hospice.

BENEFITS OF HOSPICE AND PALLIATIVE CARE

There are many benefits of palliative care within the home. It provides for familiar surroundings and more access to loved ones or pets, less exposure to institutional complications such as infections, and more patient and family control of the dying process. The physician overseeing home care must be skilled in managing pain and other symptoms and must be able to recognize psychological, spiritual and other suffering.

House calls can be highly beneficial as the physician's presence can provide the patient and family emotional and psychological support. A trusted physician can help guide identification and clarification of end-of-life goals and help them access needed community resources.

The physician may also choose to turn the care completely over to the hospice medical director and hospice team. This should not be seen as abandonment but rather as providing for the best care if the physician does not feel comfortable overseeing hospice care. Should patients require more intense services than can be provided in their home environment, hospices have contracts with local

TABLE 2 What patients and families value in hospice care

➤ Explicit support for the family so the patient feels like less of a burden

➤ Case management services

➤ Experience with the issues and programs for end-of-life care

➤ Provision of all medications, supplies, and services related to the terminal illness

➤ Support to allow the patient to leave positive legacies and good memories

➤ Having financial and other affairs in order so as not to be a burden after death

TABLE 3 Why physicians refer patients for hospice care

➤ Better care of the patient and family, including more resources to carry out the care

➤ Fewer urgent telephone calls and emergency department visits

➤ More satisfied patients and families

hospitals or nursing homes for caregiver respite or for an inpatient stay to better monitor and manage symptoms. Some hospices have a free-standing inpatient hospice. This can be used during the last few days or weeks of life if dying at home is not consistent with goals of care for the patient or family.

PHYSICIAN ROLES IN HOME HOSPICE

The hospice medical director (or hospice physician interdisciplinary team leader) is responsible for medical oversight of each individual patient's plan of care and assures that the certification of the patient for hospice services is appropriate. At the direction of the attending physician, the hospice medical director may assume complete care of the patient or may collaborate on symptom management with the attending physician. The medical director attends interdisciplinary team meetings and guides the team in implementation of the treatment plan.

The attending physician generally plays the most significant role in determining and delivering the patient's care. He or she may also be the hospice director. The attending physician must sign the initial certification and continue to see the patient as medically necessary. He or she may work with the hospice to prescribe appropriate comfort measures, and review the patient's condition and prognosis, and is responsible for the death certificate. Designation of an alternate physician for a planned absence by the attending physician is required.

TABLE 4 Attending physician responsibilities when certifying the need for hospice care

➤ Signing the initial certification for terminal illness

➤ Reviewing the hospice plan of care

➤ Making ongoing visits with the patient and caring for all medical needs

➤ Prescribing medication for comfort care

➤ Reviewing care with hospice staff

Hospice nurses are skilled in assessment of symptoms and in educating patients and families on end-stage disease processes. They visit the patient as needed and are the first responders to urgent needs. In most states they can pronounce death for hospice patients. Some hospices employ nurse practitioners and their services may be reimbursed by Medicare. A nurse practitioner may serve as the attending provider but cannot certify the patient for hospice services or serve as the hospice medical director. Physician assistants are excluded from serving as the attending provider, but they may continue to see patients as part of the home care team and bill under Medicare Part B.

Direct care aides provide assistance with activities of daily living and often much needed respite for caregivers. Therapists may be used for alleviation of symptoms by teaching proper transfers, recommending appropriate durable medical equipment, splinting, and other services. Social workers ensure that the client is receiving the benefits to which they are entitled and can provide some counseling services. Hospice chaplains offer spiritual consolation and are specially trained in the care of the dying. While they may seem superfluous to those who have their own spiritual advisors, many patients have unmet spiritual needs. Hospice chaplains can assist them to relieve suffering associated with concerns about meaning and the afterlife that may be as painful as physical suffering. Volunteers may provide companionship, run errands, or do other services. They are an essential component in relieving caregiver burden.

THE MEDICARE HOSPICE BENEFIT

The hospice benefit is contained within Medicare Part A and is the only benefit that patients may initiate without physician involvement. However, the physician must certify that life expectancy is less than six months if the patient's disease process follows its usual course. The physician should not delay hospice referral because of prognostic uncertainty. The hospice medical director can provide guidance and there is no penalty for continuing the benefit beyond the expected time, as long as further decline occurs and the patient still qualifies.

It is common for patients to improve initially with hospice services as unmet needs are addressed. A study found that lung cancer patients receiving aggressive palliation of symptoms actually lived longer and with better quality of life than those who received usual care.[1] See Table 5 for common misperceptions about hospice care that can lead to a delay in starting hospice.

The initial hospice certification is for 90 days, which may be followed by an additional 90-day period. Subsequent certifications are for 60 days. The patient's attending physician (if one exists) and hospice medical director (or hospice physician interdisciplinary team leader) must both complete the initial certification of terminal illness. No one other than a medical doctor or doctor of osteopathy can certify or recertify a terminal illness. Nurse practitioners may not certify the patient's terminal illness even if they will be serving as the patient's attending. There have been two recent additional Medicare requirements for the certification/recertification process. On October 1, 2009, Medicare added the physician narrative requirement to the certification of terminal illness. The brief, written narrative should explain the clinical findings that support a life expectancy of six months or less if the patient's disease process follows its usual course. For further details and examples of physician narratives see www.nhpco.org/files/public/regulatory/Cert-recert_tip_sheet.pdf. The second requirement began January 1, 2011, and calls for a hospice physician or nurse practitioner to have a face-to-face encounter with each hospice patient to determine continued eligibility for hospice care prior to the 180th-day recertification and each subsequent recertification, and attest that such a visit took place.

Unfortunately, many patients do not receive the full benefits of hospice as the median length of care is only about 20 days and over half of patients die in the first two weeks. Patients and families may be reluctant to accept services because they believe they are "giving up," may not wish to change home health providers, or may not be aware of the availability of the program for noncancer patients. The most common complaint from patients and families is that they were not referred sooner.

TABLE 5 Misperceptions about hospice care[2]

> ➤ Prognostic certainty that patient will die in six months is required

> ➤ Referral equals giving up "hope"

> ➤ No life-prolonging efforts may be considered while the patient is enrolled in hospice

> ➤ The patient must have a do not resuscitate (DNR) order to receive hospice

> ➤ It is uncomfortable to talk with the patient and family about hospice

> ➤ It is Medicare fraud or abuse if the patient survives beyond the certification period

> ➤ The patient can use up his or her hospice benefit if started too early

Patients must elect the Medicare hospice benefit for the terminal illness rather than traditional Medicare Part A coverage. They may still be hospitalized for nonhospice-related problems such as an acute fracture. They can choose to return to usual care and regular Part A coverage at any time, but they must revoke hospice in writing. The hospice receives a per diem from Medicare from which it must meet the needs of the patient including medications related to the hospice diagnosis and for comfort care. The hospice must also provide needed durable medical equipment such as a hospital bed or oxygen.

BILLING AND HOSPICE

Reimbursement for physician services is dependent on the role of the physician at the time of service and can be somewhat complicated. If the physician is an employee of the hospice, the hospice is billed for professional, administrative and technical services for everything associated with the hospice diagnosis. The hospice bills Medicare for the physician's professional services. If the medical director is also the patient's attending physician and services are completely unrelated to the hospice diagnosis he or she would bill Medicare directly using the "GW" modifier.

If the primary attending physician is not a hospice employee, he or she bills Medicare Part B directly for nonhospice diagnoses using the "GV" modifier. The attending may also bill for care plan oversight. Technical services, such as phlebotomy, should be billed to the hospice via a contractual agreement.

Consulting physicians need to have contracts with the hospice and bill the hospice for all services. Physician assistants may bill Medicare Part B for physician services rendered in accordance with state laws for physician supervision, but the hospice

TABLE 6 How to bill services for hospice patients: Primary attending physician (not hospice medical director)

➤ Bill Medicare Part B or applicable intermediary using your usual electronic system and the applicable evaluation and management (E/M) Current Procedural Terminology (CPT®) code for the service. Include the GV modifier, which indicates you are not hospice medical director.

➤ If you are authorized to give medication or perform a procedure, bill the medication and the technical component to your Part B carrier. For specific instructions, call the hospice claims specialist.

➤ You will be paid 80% of the Medicare allowable and should bill the patient or secondary insurance for the remaining 20%.

TABLE 7 How to bill services for hospice patients: Consulting (or second) physician

➤ Sign a Services Agreement with the hospice for each patient under your care.

➤ Bill the hospice with the applicable CPT® codes for both professional and technical components using the CMS 1500 form.

➤ You will be paid 100% of the Medicare allowable (minus any billing fees by the hospice) and will not bill the patient or secondary insurance for any component of the bill.

cannot bill Medicare for their professional services. Nurse practitioners may be the attending of record and bill Part B but only a physician can certify the patient for hospice.

RESOURCES

A comprehensive explanation of the hospice benefit can be found on the Centers for Medicare & Medicaid Services web site, www.cms.hhs.gov/manuals/Downloads/bp102c09.pdf

UNIPAC Series (9 Volumes), 3rd Edition. Hospice and Palliative Care Training for Physicians

EPERC: End of Life / Palliative Education Resource Center: www.eperc.mcw.edu. Hospice and palliative care educational resource.

The Hospice Association of America web site, www.hospice-america.org. Good resource for patients and caregivers.

Himelstein BP. Palliative care for infants, children, adolescents and their families. *J Pall Medication*. 2006:9(1):163–181.

REFERENCES

1. Jennifer S, Temel MD, et al. Early palliative care for patients with metastatic non–small-cell lung cancer. *N Engl J Med*. 2010:363;8733–8742.

2. Vig EK, Starks H, et al: Why don't patients enroll in hospice? Can we do anything about it? *J Gen Intern Med*. 2010;25 (October):1009–1019.

CHAPTER | TWELVE

New Tools for Your Home Care Bag: Technology Comes Home

After reading this chapter you should be able to:

1. Describe available diagnostic, therapeutic and safety technology for in-home use

2. Discuss how telehealth can impact home care

3. Discuss the challenges of using an electronic medical record in the mobile environment

The black bag full of useful tools is an iconic symbol of home health care, and in the last decade new technologies have emerged that clinicians should consider adding to their "bag of tricks." Although the value and specific indications for some of these technologies is still being defined, home care clinicians must understand how to use these technologies to assess and manage patients in a high quality, cost-effective way. This chapter provides a brief overview of technologies that can be used in the home to diagnose and monitor patients, and those that can be used to treat complex conditions such as chronic respiratory failure. In addition, the technology required for use of electronic medical records in home care medicine is described.

MONITORING TOOLS

Newer technologies that incorporate low-cost sensors and internet and telephonic communication links allow for ongoing monitoring of chronic illnesses and earlier recognition of clinically important changes in health status. Home monitoring has been implemented for a wide range of diseases, including chronic heart failure (CHF), chronic obstructive pulmonary disease (COPD), asthma, diabetes, hypertension, and many others.[1,2,3,4] See Table 1 for examples of technologies for home monitoring and diagnosis.

CHF is the prototypical illness monitored remotely in home settings. Currently available technologies enable patients to take daily measurements of weight and blood pressure, and answer questions to assess changes in signs or symptoms of a heart failure flare such as increased shortness of breath. Via telephone connection or the internet, the system forwards this information to

TABLE 1 Examples of technologies for home monitoring and diagnosis

Technology	Disease or indication
Two-way messaging devices	Any chronic illness
Scales that upload data	CHF, obesity
Blood pressure cuffs that upload data	Hypertension, CHF
Blood oxygen saturation monitors	CHF, COPD
12-Lead EKG devices integrated with computing devices	CAD, HTN, arrhythmias
Cardiac impedance (non-invasive measure of cardiac output)	CHF
Sleep studies	Sleep apnea, insomnia
Sensor arrays that monitor activity levels	Concern about frailty or falls
Medication dispensing and reminder devices	Nonadherence to medication
X-ray	CHF, pneumonia, trauma
Ultrasound	CHF, DVT, abdominal pain, leg wounds (vascular studies)
Digital camera	Wounds, skin lesions, environment documentation, copying forms, insurance cards, etc.

a health care professional (usually a nurse) who remotely monitors these data using a web-based program that analyzes changes in weight or symptomatology and alerts the physician when a change has occurred that requires follow up with the patient. Theoretically, these programs allow for management of CHF flares earlier and more effectively, with resultant reduction in admissions and reduced hospital lengths of stay and overall costs. Unfortunately, the literature is mixed, with some studies showing benefits, and others failing to demonstrate improvement in disease endpoints or cost.[5,6,7,8,9] Despite this uncertainty, many home care agencies and disease management companies continue to provide these services for selected patients who are either post-acute care discharge or at high risk for hospital admission. As limited as the evidence is to support the use of telemonitoring for CHF, it is even less developed for other chronic conditions.

Telehome care (beyond traditional audio phone services) is becoming increasingly available. Home health agencies and hospices can use videophone technology to perform visits within the skilled home health or hospice benefit. These visits may substitute for some, but not all, visits by the nurse or therapist. Physicians can use videophone and other technology to perform evaluation and management services, monitor physiological parameters, and verify function of medical equipment (e.g., pacemakers). Televisits can include telestethoscopes and high-definition cameras for diagnosis of skin lesions. With increasing speeds of connection available (e.g., through broadband internet connections), it is possible to evaluate movement disorders and ambulation remotely. The physician who plans to use or receive information from these devices must be knowledgeable not only about the diagnostic and treatment modalities, but also about the privacy risks inherent in internet communications, and must ensure that all of his or her programs are Health Insurance Portability and Accountability Act (HIPAA)-compliant.

Other technologies, such as motion sensor arrays and medication-dispensing systems also offer the ability to monitor and support activities of daily living (ADLs). Personal emergency medical alert systems that allow a person to press a button on a pendant or bracelet to summon help have existed for more than 30 years.[10] Newer systems employ sensor arrays in the walls and ceilings to monitor activity patterns and detect changes in behavior patterns as markers of change in function and health status. Even though these systems are promising, there is little literature to support their widespread use.[11]

Technologically advanced medication-dispensing and reminder systems have also been developed. These range from simple pill boxes with reminder beeps to fully automated systems that dispense pills at a certain time and alert caregivers remotely via e-mail or text message if the medication has not been taken. Although the literature on the value of these devices varies, in carefully selected patient populations they can improve medication adherence and safety. As with other aspects of home care, physicians must document the need for home-based technology at the time it is ordered and reassess its ongoing need over time.

Advances in technology also make home diagnosis easier. Automated blood pressure cuffs are an example of a tool that has been in clinicians' black bags for more than 100 years and are now easier to use by patients and clinicians alike. In addition, it is now possible to inexpensively obtain point-of-care blood tests for chemistries (e.g. CBCs, and INRs). EKG software now makes a common laptop computer into an EKG machine. Although payment for home-based testing may require complicated billing strategies, the relatively low cost of these procedures compared to a visit to an emergency department or hospitalization makes them almost a mandatory part of a house calls bag. In some cities mobile radiology services are available for home visits. These services include x-rays and ultrasounds that can be transmitted digitally for reading and interpretation.

THERAPEUTIC TECHNOLOGY DEVICES

Newer technologies also make provision of care that was previously only available in institutional or office settings obtainable in the home. (See Table 2 for a list of therapeutic technology services that can now be performed at home.) Ventilators,[12] hemodialysis machines,[13] and pumps for intravenous medications and parenteral nutrition are now widely available for patients of all ages. As with any use of these technologies, close collaboration between the physician, patient and family caregivers, and other professionals is required. For example, every patient on a ventilator will need respiratory therapy support and should also have a pulmonologist's input and consultation if possible.

Availability of higher technology devices has also led to the development of new home-based programs of care, such as hospital at home programs.[14] Over the past 20 years several programs to treat patients at home in lieu of acute hospitalization have been shown to be successful alternatives for selected patients. However, despite literature supporting the safety and efficacy of these programs, their dissemination in the United States remains limited.

TABLE 2 Examples of high technology therapeutic home care devices

Hemodialysis
Pumps for parenteral nutrition and intravenous medications
Invasive and non-invasive ventilator support devices
Pumps for enteral nutrition

ELECTRONIC MEDICAL RECORDS (EMR) IN THE MOBILE ENVIRONMENT

Despite challenges for mobile health care clinicians, many, if not most, are using electronic medical record (EMR) systems. Although a full discussion of EMRs in the mobile environment is beyond the scope of this publication, further information on the topic is available on the American Academy of Home Care Physicians web site (www.aahcp.org). The mobile medical record has three inter-related components: hardware, software, and the communications systems. The key challenge is that in a mobile environment, the clinician cannot be certain of connection to the Internet continuously, an assumption taken for granted in the wired, office-based practice. Virtually all of the modern EMR designs began with a client/server architecture, which limited the ability to share data between an internet-based server and a mobile computer without a continuous connection. Basically, the two solutions are 1) intermittent sharing of data when a connection is available; or 2) accepting that if a clinician loses a connection in the middle of transmission, a risk of incomplete or inaccurate communication exists. The former limits efficiency of communication that could delay decision-making (e.g., while awaiting access to a patient chart) or treatment (e.g., awaiting transmission of orders). The latter can lead to uncertainty about transmission of orders or the need to recreate documentation that was lost in the process.

A second issue in mobile electronic medical records is size of records. The average chart size for an EMR, according to a Federal Communications Commission report in 2010, was 5 megabytes, too large to send reliably over the types of wireless communications tools most widely available (e.g., 3G aircard). Newer systems available in large metropolitan areas offer faster communication speeds, but it is unclear when they will be available in less dense population centers.[15] Unfortunately, government incentives for use of EMRs were established without full recognition of these problems. Physicians selecting mobile EMRs are strongly encouraged by these incentives to use vendors that meet standards that require high-speed, reliable communications, but such systems either delay or risk loss of data in transmission from the mobile environment. Physicians working within a larger clinic or health system often have no choice but to use software designed for office settings. Careful consideration of the challenges and trade-offs is necessary.

The hardware choices for mobile health providers are ever expanding. Most common, based on office-based EMR models, is the traditional laptop computer that requires a seating arrangement that permits typing. Tablet computers that allow data entry on the screen are widely used in home medicine, since they permit data entry with one hand and, for some, completion of forms that require a signature. Smart phones and tablet devices routinely carried by physicians, such as those running Apple iOS (for iPad®), Android™ or WebOS operating systems, will become an increasing part of EMR tools.

There are a rapidly growing number of technology companies in the fields of assistive devices, point-of-care (POC) diagnostics, and clinical management (which includes remote patient monitoring (RPM), EMRs, and communications). A continually updated directory of such companies is available at: http://www.aahcp.org/associations/11307/files/Technology%20Companies%20of%20possible%20interest%20to%20Housecall%20Clinicians.pdf. This list is intended to provide a compilation of emerging companies that might provide strategic value with integration into house call practice settings.

CONCLUSIONS

New technologies for home monitoring and high technology care have the potential to make providing care for frail and medically complex patients at home more effective. The indications and effectiveness of many of these technologies are still being evaluated, but physicians should become familiar with these tools and incorporate them into their practices for selected patients. It should be noted that the use of technology does not relieve the physician of basic human requirements of patient care. There is no substitute for a home visit in monitoring chronic care and dealing with problems as they arise. Arrangements must be made for regular physician hands-on care of the patient who is receiving high-technology home care so that the physician can remain fully aware of the patient's health status and maintain a strong therapeutic alliance with the patient and any caregivers. Documentation of those encounters can, and probably should be, entered into the EMR system, despite challenges for such systems in the mobile environment.

REFERENCES

1. Paré G, Moqadem K, Pineau G, St-Hilaire C. Clinical effects of home telemonitoring in the context of diabetes, asthma, heart failure and hypertension: a systematic review. *J Med Internet Res.* 2010;12(2):e21.

2. Paré G, Moqadem K, Pineau G, St-Hilaire C. Clinical effects of home telemonitoring in the context of diabetes, asthma, heart failure and hypertension: a systematic review. *J Med Internet Res.* 2010;12(2):e21.

3. Jaana M, Paré G, Sicotte C. Home telemonitoring for respiratory conditions: a systematic review. *Am J Manag Care.* 2009;(5):313–320.

4. Polisena J, Tran K, Cimon K, Hutton B, McGill S, Palmer K, Scott RE. Home telemonitoring for congestive heart failure: a systematic review and meta-analysis. *J Telemed Telecare.* 2010;16(2):68–76.

5. Koehler F, Winkler S, Schieber M, Sectim U, Stangl K, Bohm M, et al. Impact of remote tele-medical management on mortality and hospitalizations in ambulatory patients with chronic heart failure: The Telemedical Interventional Monitoring in Heart Failure Study. *Circulation.* 2011;123(17):1873–1880.

6. Wakefield BJ, Ward MM, Holman JE, et al. Evaluation of home telehealth following hospitalization for heart failure: a randomized trial. *Telemed J E Health.* 2008;14(8):753–761.

7. Chaudhry SI, Mattera JA, Curtis JP, Spertus JA, et al. Telemonitoring in patients with heart failure. *N Engl J Med.* 2010;363(24):2301–2309.

8. Antonicelli R, Testarmata P, Spazzafumo L, et al. Impact of telemonitoring at home on the management of elderly patients with congestive heart failure. *J Telemed Telecare.* 2008;14(6):300–305.

9. Weintraub A, Gregory D, Patel AR, et al. A multicenter randomized controlled evaluation of automated home monitoring and telephonic disease management in patients recently hospitalized for congestive heart failure: the SPAN-CHF II trial. *J Card Fail.* 2010;16(4):285–292.

10. Ruchlin HS, Morris JN. Cost-benefit analysis of an emergency alarm and response system: a case study of a long-term care program. *Health Serv Res.* 1981;16(1):65–80.

11. Brownsell S, Bradley D, Blackburn S, Cardinaux F, Hawley MS. A systematic review of lifestyle monitoring technologies. *J Telemed Telecare.* 2011;17(4)185–189.

12. Lewarski JS, Gay PC. Current issues in home mechanical ventilation. *Chest.* 2007;132(2): 671–676.

13. Qamar M, Bender F, Rault R, Piraino B. The United States' perspectives on home dialysis. *Adv Chronic Kidney Dis.* 2009;16(3):189–197.

14. Cheng J, Montalto M, Leff B. Hospital at home. *Clin Geriatr Med.* 2009;25(1):79–91, vi.

15. Federal Communications Commission. National Broadband Plan. 2010. http://www.broadband.gov/plan/10-healthcare/. Accessed November 2011.

CHAPTER THIRTEEN

Medical Ethics in Home Care

After reading this chapter you should be able to:

1. Discuss the American Medical Association (AMA) Principles of Medical Ethics subsections that are applicable and have been modified to apply to physicians involved in home care

2. Recognize fraudulent home care practices

PRINCIPLES

Home care involves a wide spectrum of participants and occurs in a venue that is beyond the physician's direct control. It is important, therefore, to understand ethical issues and pitfalls when applying a home-based approach to patient care. The following are each of the American Medical Association (AMA) Principles of Medical Ethics[1] subsections that are applicable and have been modified to apply to physicians involved in home care.

AMA PRINCIPLES OF MEDICAL ETHICS

Preamble

The medical profession has long subscribed to a body of ethical statements developed primarily for the benefit of the patient. As a member of this profession, a physician must recognize responsibility not only to patients but also to society, to other health professionals, and to self. The following principles, adopted by the AMA, are not laws, but standards of conduct which define the essentials of honorable behavior for the physician.

Section 1

A physician shall be dedicated to providing competent medical service with compassion and respect for human dignity.

1. The home care physician will respect the dignity and privacy of the patient and the patient's home.

2. The home care physician will be vigilant regarding the physical and emotional boundaries of the doctor/patient relationship.

3. The home care physician will not be a party to any type of policy that excludes, segregates, or demeans the dignity of any patient because of ethnic origin, race, sex, creed, age, socioeconomic status, or sexual orientation.

Section 2

A physician shall deal honestly with patients and colleagues, and strive to expose those physicians deficient in character or competence, or who engage in fraud or deception.

1. The home care physician will practice and provide services within his/her usual area of competence, exclusive of emergent needs.

2. The home care physician will explicitly establish the terms of the financial arrangements with the patient.

3. Payment to physicians by home health agencies must be compensation for appropriate activities and must not be provided as an inducement for referrals.

4. Physician referrals for home health agency services, home diagnostics, home medical equipment, and other non-physician home care services will be determined by legitimate clinical needs and will not be motivated by personal gain or self-interest.

5. Physicians practicing in the home care setting will be honest and forthright with patients, informing them of any factors that may affect their care, including, but not limited to, expectations and/or changes regarding visit frequency, identity of who will be rendering the care, and the relationship of that individual to a medical group or organization, if not in solo practice.

Section 3

A physician shall respect the law and also recognize a responsibility to seek changes in those requirements which are contrary to the best interests of the patient.

1. The home care physician will request payment only for those services rendered.

2. The home care physician will render only those services indicated by the circumstances of the clinical setting.

3. Specifically, those physicians ordering patient services or supplies from a home health agency will be responsible for timely approval of the care plan and subsequent orders, including service lines involved (occupational therapy, physical therapy, etc.), frequency of home visits, and medications.

4. A physician who requests payment for Care Plan Oversight is expected to have provided the services detailed within the guidelines and regulations provided by the payer source.

Section 4

A physician shall respect the rights of the patient, of colleagues, and of other healing professionals, and shall safeguard patient confidences within the constraints of the law.

1. The home care physician will protect the patient's confidentiality as expected in a patient/physician relationship with special attention to protecting records or other pertinent information from public exposure, for example, within view in the physician's automobile.

2. The home care physician may release confidential information only with the authorization of the patient or under proper legal compulsion.

3. The home care physician will respect the advance directives already established or seek clarity from the patient or appropriate family member when no clear directive has been prepared.

Section 5

A physician shall continue to study, apply, and advance scientific knowledge, make relevant information available to patients, colleagues, and the public, obtain consultation, and use the talents of other health professionals when indicated.

1. In view of rapid development of technological advances affecting medical care provided in the home, the home care physician will be responsible for his/her own continuing education and be mindful that theirs must be a lifetime of learning.

2. The home care physician will often be involved with providers of services from a variety of fields. The home care physician needs to recognize both his/her role in the leadership and direction of the patient's care and his/her role in facilitating the activities of the other providers.

3. When possible, the home care physician will provide education and/or consultative services to home health agency personnel, so as to encourage continual learning and improvement in clinical skills.

Section 6

A physician shall, in the provision of appropriate patient care, except in emergencies, be free to choose whom to service, with whom to associate, and the environment in which to provide medical services.

1. The home care physician will determine whether or not the home is the appropriate environment in which to diagnose and treat the patient.

2. The home care physician may refuse to provide treatment to a person who, in the physician's opinion, cannot be adequately evaluated in the home setting.

3. The home care physician has a right to determine if entering a neighborhood or specific domicile is safe. If determined or suspected to be unsafe, the physician has the right to decline the home visit. A physician who declines to make a visit under these circumstances has an obligation to communicate with the patient/caregiver and arrange for an alternative approach to care for the patient.

Section 7

A physician shall recognize a responsibility to participate in activities contributing to an improved community.

1. Home care physicians are encouraged to communicate and cooperate with health care and government organizations in order to promote an improved environment for the practice of medicine in the home.

2. Physicians with home care experience are encouraged to teach their colleagues about treating patients in the home setting, convey their experience, and establish techniques that provide for a safe and secure environment for the practice of medicine.

3. Physicians will respect the professional integrity and needs of non-physicians on the home care team and will interact with these others in an appropriate manner commensurate with that professional respect.

RECOGNIZING FRAUDULENT PRACTICES

Unscrupulous suppliers and providers may steer physicians into signing or authorizing improper certifications of medical necessity.[2] The Office of the Inspector General (OIG) of the U.S. Department of Health and Human Services has identified home health care and hospice as vulnerable to fraud and abuse.[3] Medicare requires physicians to play a key role in determining the medical need and utilization of home health care. The Medicare program relies on the professional judgment of the patient's treating physician to authorize services from home health agencies (HHAs) and products from medical equipment suppliers.

AVOID PARTICIPATING IN FRAUDULENT PRACTICES

The OIG's Operation Restore Trust audit in 1997 identified four main classes of abusive practices involving home health DME agencies:[4]

➤ Unnecessary visits and services were provided

➤ Patients were not homebound

➤ There were no valid physician orders

➤ There was insufficient documentation

Of the physicians who signed plans of care for unallowable claims, 64% relied on the HHA to prepare the plan of care, 60% were not aware of the homebound requirement for home services, and 8% had no knowledge of the patient's condition.[5]

HOW TO MANAGE CERTIFICATIONS FOR HOME HEALTH AGENCY SERVICES

Knowing the patient and examining the plan of care (Home Health Certification and Plan of Care, which can be completed on Centers for Medicare & Medicaid Services (CMS) form 485 or a similar document) are crucial to the physician's

TABLE 1 Strategies to avoid fostering or participating in home health fraud

> ➤ Learn the basic coverage guidelines for home health care and durable medical equipment (DME).

> ➤ Never sign the HHA "Home Health Certification and Plan of Care" for patients who are clearly not homebound. (Note: the Medicare definition of homebound allows the HHA to service a wide range of patients—see Chapter 4 for the definition of "homebound.")

> ➤ Never sign a blank certificate of medical necessity for DME.

> ➤ Never accept compensation in exchange for your signature. Such compensation can take the form of cash payments; free goods, services or products offered below fair market value; and rental of space offered below fair market value.

> ➤ If you cannot provide house calls to your homebound patients to determine the appropriateness of DME, consider making a referral to a consulting physician who specializes in home care (a home care consultant).

ability to minimize the risk for fraud. The physician should not sign the care plan without first reviewing its contents. Effective April 2011 a physician who certifies a patient as eligible for Medicare home health services must see the patient face to face and document how the patient's clinical condition supports a homebound status and the need for skilled services (see Chapter 2 and http://www.cms.gov/MLNMattersArticles/downloads/SE1038.pdf).

DURABLE MEDICAL EQUIPMENT (DME)

Medicare covers DME (e.g., hospital beds, wheelchairs, home oxygen), prosthetics, orthotics, and supplies for home care use. As a condition for payment, Medicare requires the treating physician to provide a signed prescription,

TABLE 2 Red flags for abusive durable medical equipment (DME) authorization requests

> ➤ Frequent requests from a particular vendor or provider to sign for devices or services that you did not order

> ➤ Added features on DME orders (e.g., deluxe or electric features on a wheelchair)

> ➤ High-frequency tests or test results not reported (e.g., home glucose or INR monitoring)

and medical equipment must be prescribed only by physicians. For certain equipment and supplies, the prescription takes the form of a certificate of medical necessity (CMN). The physician should not allow a DME company to specify what equipment to order for the patient. Medical equipment or supplies can be prescribed by physicians, nurse practitioners and physician assistants. Before signing prescriptions and CMNs, the physician must always review the contents and be alert for additions to the original order. Also, he or she must confirm that what was ordered was delivered. For example, if a humidifier was ordered in conjunction with prescribing home oxygen, the patient or caregivers should confirm that it was provided. It is also illegal for DME companies to make unsolicited telephone calls to Medicare beneficiaries. Because of fraud in this area the OIG in January 2010 reiterated the illegality of DME telemarketing by issuing an updated special fraud alert, "Telemarketing by Durable Medical Equipment Suppliers."[6]

PAYING OR RECEIVING KICKBACKS IN EXCHANGE FOR MEDICARE OR MEDICAID REFERRALS

Physicians need to carefully examine financial relationships with providers of home care services. Under the anti-kickback statute, "it is illegal to knowingly and willfully solicit, receive, offer or pay anything of value to induce, or in return for, referring, recommending or arranging for the furnishing of any item or service payable by Medicare or Medicaid."[3] It is important to keep the original intent of the anti-kickback statute in mind, as it provides broad powers for claims against physicians engaged in otherwise legal activities.

TABLE 3 Examples of kickbacks that the OIG has prosecuted

➤ Payment of a fee to a physician for each plan of care certified by the physician on behalf of the home health agency.

➤ Disguising referral fees as salaries by paying referring physicians for services not rendered or in excess of fair market value for the service

➤ Offering free services to patients, including transportation and meals, if they agree to switch home health providers

➤ Providing hospitals with discharge planners, home care coordinators, or home care liaisons in order to induce referrals

➤ Providing free services, such as 24-hour nursing coverage, to retirement homes or adult congregate living facilities in return for home health referrals

➤ Marketing uncovered or unneeded home care services to patients

In addition, recent investigations have applied the anti-racketeering laws (RICO) to press criminal charges against physicians for participating in a scam to defraud the federal government. Under the RICO statutes, the Department of Justice does not need to prove a physician even knew he or she was involved or knew that the arrangement was illegal. This standard of participation —"knowingly or unknowingly" — in an illegal arrangement can be dangerous for a physician who might believe that "looking the other way" is adequate protection.

The general ethical guidelines for physicians involved in home care are presented in Table 4.

TABLE 4 Protecting yourself and your patients

➤ Never sign a home health plan of care or a certificate of medical necessity (CMN) for home equipment for a patient for whose care you are not responsible. While you are taking calls or covering for another physician, you may have the responsibility for those patients' care needs, including their home care. Having access to current chart information may be critical.

➤ Before you sign a Medicare home health plan of care, be certain that the patient meets eligibility requirements (through your own observations and knowledge of the patient or through discussions with the patient and home health agency staff).

➤ Read the home health plan of care, double-checking not only the diagnosis and medications but also the services provided and their frequencies.

➤ If you have any doubts, contact the agency and ask for clarification about why the services are necessary.

➤ Correct any errors you find on the home health plan of care or CMN and initial any corrections before you sign it.

➤ Discuss with the patient and family the limited nature of the Medicare home health benefit and the fact that they may need to find and pay for additional home care services. Provide them with information about community resources.

➤ While the patient is receiving home health services, periodically discuss with the patient and family whether these services are occurring, whether they are satisfied with the care, whether they can see they are making progress, and how long they feel the services will be needed. If they identify continuing long-term care needs beyond Medicare or other insurance coverage, talk to the HHA social worker about arranging for community resources.

➤ If home medical equipment has been ordered, periodically check for continuing use and need.

➤ While the patient is receiving home health services, request periodic written reports from the agency verifying the patient's continued homebound status and eligibility for Medicare or other home health benefits.

REPORTING HOME CARE FRAUD AND ABUSE

To report suspected home health care or Medicare fraud, call the U.S. Office of the Inspector General at (800) 447-8477 or send an e-mail to *HHSTips@oig .hhs.gov.*

REFERENCES

1. American Medical Association Code of Medical Ethics. American Medical Association web site. http://www.ama-assn.org/ama/pub/physician-resources/medical-ethics/code-medical-ethics/principles-medical-ethics.page Accessed September 23, 2011.

2. Office of Inspector General, U.S. Dept of Health and Human Services. Special Fraud Alert: Physician Liability for Certifications in the Provision of Medical Equipment and Supplies and Home Health Services. January 1999. http://oig.hhs.gov/fraud/docs/alertsandbulletins/dme.htm. Accessed September 23, 2011.

3. Office of Inspector General, U.S. Dept of Health and Human Services. *Results of the Operation Restore Trust Audit of Medicare Home. http://www.oig.hhs.gov/oas/reports/region4/49602121.pdf.* Accessed September 23, 2011.

4. Office of Inspector General, U.S. Dept of Health and Human Services. Results of the Operation Restore Trust Audit of Medicare Home Health Services in California, Illinois, New York and Texas. July 1997. http://oig.hhs.gov/oas/reports/region4/49602121.pdf. Accessed September 23, 2011.

5. Office of Inspector General, U.S .Dept of Health and Human Services. *Home Health: Problem Providers and Their Impact on Medicare.* July 1997. http://oig.hhs.gov/oei/reports/oei-09-96-00110.pdf. Accessed September 23, 2011.

6. Office of Inspector General, U.S .Dept of Health and Human Services. *Updated Special Fraud Alert: Telemarketing by Durable Medical Equipment Suppliers.* January 2010. http://oig.hhs.gov/fraud/docs/alertsandbulletins/fraudalert_telemarketing.pdf. Accessed September 23, 2011.

CHAPTER | FOURTEEN

A Patient's Rights and Responsibilities

After reading this chapter you should be able to:

1. Identify patients' rights and responsibilities per Medicare's home health condition of participation

Patients receiving in-home services and their caregivers possess certain basic rights and bear particular responsibilities. The patient is in control of many aspects of health care rendered in his or her home. With that control, concomitant responsibilities arise that must be met if the patient is to achieve the desired health care benefits.

TABLE 1 Patient's rights

> ➤ Be treated with dignity and consideration, respect, and timely attention to his or her needs

> ➤ Have his or her property treated with respect

> ➤ Have confidentiality of all information related to care within required regulations

> ➤ Be fully informed of the care and treatment that will be provided by the physician and others, how much it will cost, how payments will be handled, and whether the patient is responsible for any of those payments

> ➤ Discuss benefits, risks, and costs of appropriate treatment alternatives with the physician

> ➤ Receive guidance from his or her physicians as to their recommended course of treatment

(Continued)

TABLE 1 *Continued*

➤ Be advised of potential conflicts of interest that physicians may have, and of the right to receive independent professional opinions

➤ Have freedom of choice in care providers, to receive care from professionally competent personnel, and to know the names and responsibilities of people giving the care

➤ Have the option to accept or refuse treatment or forms of health care recommended by the physician, and to be informed of the consequences of this action

➤ Participate actively in the design of a care plan, and help update it as needs change

➤ Receive training in all aspects of self-care

➤ Experience continuity in the home care provided

➤ Be informed by a home health agency (HHA) of any anticipated termination of agency service and be referred elsewhere

➤ Have the freedom to make a complaint or recommend changes in services, or in agency policy, and to know how to do so

➤ Exercise his or her rights as a patient of the HHA

➤ Voice grievances regarding treatment or care that is (or fails to be) furnished, or regarding lack of respect for property by anyone who is furnishing services

➤ Be informed in advance about the care to be furnished, and of any changes in the care to be furnished

➤ Have confidentiality of the clinical records maintained by the HHA

➤ Be informed in advance about payment—what will be reimbursed by Medicare or other sources, and what may be required from the patient

➤ Be advised of the availability of the toll-free HHA hotline(s) (numbers vary by state)

TABLE 2 Patient's responsibilities

➤ Remain under a physician's care while receiving home care services

➤ Inform the home care team of any changes in physicians involved in the patient's care

➤ Provide the physician and the agency with a complete and accurate health history

➤ Provide the physician and the agency with all requested insurance and financial information

➤ Sign the required consents and releases for insurance billing

➤ Provide a safe home environment in which care can be given; allow necessary changes in the home environment

➤ Cooperate with the physician, the agency staff, and other caregivers by complying with the agreed upon therapy

➤ Accept responsibility for refusal of treatment

➤ Treat the physician and other health professionals with respect and consideration

➤ Advise the physician or agency administrator of any dissatisfaction or concerns about the care provided

➤ Provide physician name of Power of Attorney for Health Care

➤ Inform the physician/agency of medical appointments, hospitalizations, changes in residence, or other reasons why the patient will not be home for scheduled visits

GENERAL REFERENCE

Information is this chapter was adapted in part from information in 42 CFR 484.10 (Code of Federal Regulations)-Condition of participation: Patient rights. http://www.cms.gov/manuals/Downloads/som107ap_b_hha.pdf

CHAPTER FIFTEEN

Detection and Treatment of Elder and Child Abuse and Neglect in Home Care

After reading this chapter you should be able to:

1. Determine what constitutes elder abuse, the different types of elder abuse and how to detect them

2. Recognize the characteristics of abusers

3. Describe what constitutes self-neglect and how home care can help

4. Explain mandatory reporting and how to work with adult protective services

5. Identify what constitutes child abuse, mandatory reporting and how to help

Mistreatment of elders and people with disabilities is often hard to detect and difficult to deal with when detected (see Table 1). Victims often fear reporting abuse for several reasons. They may fear family embarrassment and humiliation or that greater abuse may occur. Frequently, they fear the loss of their caregiver and subsequent placement in a nursing home. Physicians may not be aware of or detect the signs of abuse and may be reluctant to report suspected abuse. This is due in part to a lack of standard reporting guidelines, support services, and intervention strategies for victims such as counseling and shelters. There has also been a lack of treatment options for the abusers. Finally, societal ambivalence toward the aged and disabled has played a role. One result is that research on elder abuse has lagged behind research into other forms of abuse such as child and domestic abuse. Studies of the prevalence of elder mistreatment have varied widely, but it is estimated that between 1 and 2 million Americans aged 65 years and older suffer some form of mistreatment.

Estimated frequency of elder abuse ranges from 2% to 10% based on various sampling, survey methods and case definitions.[1] Data on elder abuse in domestic settings suggest that 1 in 14 incidents, excluding incidents of self-neglect, come to the attention of authorities.[2] Elder mistreatment is associated with increased morbidity and mortality.[3] Home care including physician house calls offers a unique opportunity to uncover this often hidden problem (see Table 2).

TABLE 1 Types of elder abuse and abuse of people with disabilities

➤ Physical abuse: intentional infliction of injury or physical mistreatment, restraint, confinement and under or over use of medication

➤ Sexual abuse: any nonconsensual sexual contact (Note: Any sexual contact between a facility staff person, such as in a nursing home or assisted living facility, and a vulnerable adult is considered nonconsensual.)

➤ Psychological: includes intimidation, coercion, harassment, ridicule, isolation from family or friends, yelling or swearing

➤ Financial: illegal or improper use of the property, resources, or income of a vulnerable elder for another person's profit or gain

➤ Neglect: Can be passive, active or self-neglect

TABLE 2 Evidence of elder abuse is most easily obtained during a home visit

➤ Physical abuse may result in bruises in different stages of healing, rope burns or bruises around the wrists, axillae or ankles from restraints, pressure sores and cigarette burns. Sexual abuse constitutes less than 1% of reported cases of elder mistreatment.[4] Signs include genital or urinary irritation, injury or scarring. Unlike in child abuse, fractures of the long bones or ribs in the elderly are more often pathologic rather than signs of abuse. Recurrent cancellations of home care visits should alert the physician to the potential for abuse.

➤ Verbal and emotional abuse may be suspected if a patient demonstrates fear or hostility in the presence of the caregiver. It takes the form of name-calling, threats such as possible nursing home placement, and isolation from activities.

➤ Misappropriation of finances may be signaled by the absence of prescribed medications or supplies. Persuading an elder to part with money is the most common form of financial abuse. Other forms of financial abuse include getting elders to change their wills or sign over their homes or other assets.

➤ Neglect is sometimes manifested as poor hygiene, inadequate nutrition, or non-compliance with medications. However, it is important not to over-interpret these findings, as some patients may refuse to eat or take their medications, or resist treatments or personal attention.

Elder neglect is classified into passive, active, and self-neglect. Passive neglect exists when a need is inadvertently unmet or a risk is unintentionally created because the caregiver is unaware or incapable of meeting the elder's needs. Victims of passive neglect often require a high level of care and tend to be mentally and physically disabled. The caregiver or elder or both may be unable or unwilling to accept or pay for necessary services. Alternatively, community resources may not be available. Active neglect is when the caregiver knowingly and maliciously does not meet the elder's needs. Self-neglect is when the elder fails to perform or acquire services necessary to maintain his or her health and well-being. Self-neglect is the most common type of mistreatment, representing nearly half of all cases reported to adult protective services (APS) and is often the most difficult to deal with when identified.[5] Self-neglect is not revealed by many screens but can be readily apparent on a home visit. Signs of elder neglect include body odor, decayed teeth, soiled clothing and bedding, pressure sores, and an unsafe living environment.

Initial research on elder abusers focused on the burden and stress of caregiving. Caregivers often become isolated as they focus more time on meeting the needs of the elder and forgo time for themselves. Caregivers frequently have little respite, and their work often goes unnoticed and unrecognized. Elder characteristics that increase caregiver stress include requiring high levels of physical and emotional care and the troublesome behaviors that come with dementia. These behaviors include wandering, repeating questions, leaving stoves and ovens on, and attacking caregivers physically and verbally. It has been found that the emotional burden rather than the physical work is the greatest stress to caregivers. The term "caregiver stress" must be used discriminately so it does not allow for victim-blaming of the elder and prevent the abuser from being held accountable. While caregiver stress is involved in elder mistreatment, more recent research identifies other abuser characteristics as more significant.[6] These include financial and emotional dependency on the elder, alcohol abuse, substance abuse, history of violent behavior, and psychiatric problems (mainly depression). Abuser characteristics, rather than elder characteristics, are more predictive of elder mistreatment.

Elder mistreatment is considered a major health issue by The Joint Commission and the American Medical Association. The home care population is a subgroup of elders particularly at risk for mistreatment; therefore, screening is recommended by many. Separate interviews with the patient and abuser are helpful in diagnosing elder mistreatment. See Table 3 for screening questions for the patient. Any physical signs of abuse or neglect as listed above should be clearly documented.

When interviewing the alleged abuser it can be helpful to use the label "unmet needs" of the elder rather than the more emotionally charged words of "abuse" or "neglect". The focus should be on the common goal of quality care for the elder and a desire to obtain the services necessary for this care (see Table 4).

TABLE 3 Abuse screening questions for the patient

➤ Do you feel safe? If not, why?

➤ Is anyone hurting you? Have you ever been shoved, shaken, hit or restrained against your will?

➤ Are your needs being met and in a timely fashion?

➤ Have you ever been threatened, ridiculed or asked to do something against your will?

➤ Do you have any fears about how your money is being spent? Has any of your money or property been taken or signed over to someone else?

➤ Is your caregiver dependent on you financially? Does your caregiver have any history of violent behavior, alcohol abuse, drug abuse or mental disorder including depression?

TABLE 4 Questions for the alleged abuser

➤ Tell me about the elder you care for. What kind of care does he or she require?

➤ What can the elder do for him or herself?

➤ What does the elder expect from you? Are you able to do what the elder expects?

➤ What are your responsibilities outside the home?

➤ Caring for an elder can be a very difficult task. Have you ever felt so frustrated that you pushed, hit or slapped the elder? What were the circumstances?

➤ Have there been times when you have yelled at or threatened the elder?

➤ What services would help support you in taking care of the elder?

The first determination to make when elder mistreatment is suspected is whether there is immediate danger to the elder. If possible danger exists, 911 or APS should be called immediately. If there is not any immediate danger, states vary as to reporting requirements (to see state reporting requirements go to www.abanet.ogr/aging/docs/MandatoryReportingProvisionsChart.pdf). Reporting elder mistreatment is mandatory for health care workers in the majority of states; however, the resources for handling these reports and the penalties for failure to report vary widely (there is no federal standard). Most statutes include a "good Samaritan" clause whereby a person reporting abuse cannot face legal action if he or she has done so in good faith and without malicious intent or for personal profit. Health care providers should know the law and reporting requirements for their state. This information can also be obtained from the local APS program or the local or state Department on Aging. Physicians may be reluctant to file reports with APS because they fear adding burdens to already overwhelmed caregivers who have good intentions. In most states, legislation now exists that stipulates a social service professional make the first investigative contact with the elder and family (see Table 5). Reporting to APS can thus be presented to the elder and caregiver as another resource for obtaining added support. A competent patient has the right to refuse protective services.

Any interventions need to be pursued in a multidisciplinary manner and will most likely be coordinated by APS. The solution ideally should be the least restrictive to the elder and all attempts should be made to keep the patient at home in order to preserve patient autonomy. The first determination for intervention is to learn if the elder is willing to accept help and support services. If willing, then he or she should be educated about elder mistreatment and the tendency for it to increase over time. A plan is then implemented to insure the elder's safety. Support, education and treatment for the abuser should be set up. The availability and cost of community resources including homemaker, counseling, legal and financial services should be made known to the patient. If the patient is unwilling to receive intervention, then a determination of mental capacity needs to be made. If the elder has capacity and refuses intervention, he or she should be educated that the severity and frequency of elder mistreatment may increase in the future. The patient should have written instructions regarding emergency numbers and a safety plan. Follow-up care needs to be determined and discussed with the patient. If the patient is unwilling to accept help but is found to lack capacity, varying degrees of legal action can be undertaken. The legal process can be minimal, such as direct deposit of checks with a representative payee, or more extensive such as obtaining guardianship. Rarely does the criminal justice system need to become involved, but legal actions can be taken against the abuser, ranging from a protection order to imprisonment.

TABLE 5 Adult protective services' interventions include, but are not limited to

---

➤ Receiving reports of elder/vulnerable adult abuse, neglect, and/or exploitation

➤ Investigating reports and collecting evidence

➤ Assessing the victim's risk

➤ Assessing the victim's capacity to understand his or her risk and ability to give informed consent

➤ Developing a case plan

➤ Arranging for services, including respite

➤ Service monitoring

➤ Pursuing legal action if necessary

CHILD ABUSE

Child abuse involves doing something or failing to do something that results in harm to a child or puts a child at risk of harm. Child abuse can be physical, sexual or emotional. Neglect, or not providing for a child's needs, is also considered to be a form of abuse. Munchausen's by proxy syndrome is a unique form of abuse where a parent or caregiver misleads others into thinking that the child has medical problems by deliberately creating or exaggerating the child's symptoms in several ways. These individuals might lie, falsify medical records, or induce symptoms by giving the child medicine or toxic substances. As a result, doctors usually order tests, try different types of medications, and may even hospitalize the child or perform unnecessary surgery.

Most child abuse occurs within the family, often committed by parents or relatives who themselves were abused as children. Neglect and mistreatment of children is also more common in families living in poverty and among parents who are teenagers or are drug or alcohol abusers. According to a 2007 U.S. Department of Health and Human Services, Administration for Children and Families report, child protective services (CPS) agencies received nearly 3.2 million reports of child maltreatment.[7] The current economic recession is also having a negative effect, with many states imposing budget cuts that affect child welfare programs. Inadequate resources are stretching state child protection agencies too thin to properly serve at-risk children and their families.

CHILDREN WITH SPECIAL HEALTH CARE NEEDS

Most parents, foster parents, and caregivers take exceptional care of children with special health care needs, especially when they are technology dependent or are being treated at home for a wide variety of acquired or congenital medical, developmental, or other mental health problems. However, children with disabilities are the most likely to suffer abuse and may be more at risk because of parent or caregiver stress and frustration in caring for them combined with being more vulnerable because of their disability. Lack of caregiver knowledge and ability along with inadequate community supports also contribute.

Children, especially those with developmental disabilities, may not report abuse because they do not understand what abuse is or what acts are abusive. Communication problems may also make it difficult for children to understand and talk about episodes of abuse.[8]

Each state is responsible for providing its own definitions of child abuse and neglect. Most states recognize four major types of maltreatment: neglect, physical abuse, sexual abuse, and emotional abuse. Although any of the forms of child maltreatment may be found separately, they often occur in combination. The examples provided below are for general informational purposes only. Not all states' definitions will include all of the listed examples and individual states' definitions may cover additional situations not mentioned here.

Neglect is failure to provide for a child's basic needs. Neglect may be:

➤ Physical (e.g., failure to provide necessary food or shelter, or lack of appropriate supervision)

➤ Medical (e.g., failure to provide necessary medical or mental health treatment)

➤ Educational (e.g., failure to educate a child or attend to special education needs)

➤ Emotional (e.g., inattention to a child's emotional needs, failure to provide psychological care, or permitting the child to use alcohol or other drugs)

These situations do not always mean a child is neglected. Sometimes cultural values, the standards of care in the community, and poverty may be contributing factors, indicating the family is in need of information or assistance. When a family fails to use information and resources, and the child's health or safety is at risk, then child welfare intervention may be required.

Physical abuse is physical injury (ranging from minor bruises to severe fractures or death) as a result of punching, beating, kicking, biting, shaking, throwing, stabbing, choking, hitting (with a hand, stick, strap, or other object), burning, or otherwise harming a child. Such injury is considered abuse regardless of whether the caretaker intended to hurt the child.

Sexual abuse includes activities by a parent or caretaker such as fondling a child's genitals, penetration, incest, rape, sodomy, indecent exposure, and exploitation through prostitution or the production of pornographic materials.

Emotional abuse is a pattern of behavior that impairs a child's emotional development or sense of self-worth. This may include constant criticism, threats, or rejection, as well as withholding love, support, or guidance. Emotional abuse is often difficult to prove and, therefore, CPS may not be able to intervene without evidence of harm to the child. Emotional abuse is almost always present when other forms of abuse are identified.

REPORTING CHILD ABUSE OR NEGLECT

All 50 states, the District of Columbia, and the U.S. Territories have enacted statutes specifying procedures that a mandatory reporter must follow when making a report of child abuse or neglect. Mandatory reporters are individuals who are required by law to report cases of suspected child abuse or neglect. In most states, the statutes require mandated reporters to make a report immediately after gaining their knowledge or suspicion of abusive or neglectful situations. In all jurisdictions, the initial report may be made orally to either the CPS agency or to a law enforcement agency. For a listing of mandated reporters, see Department of Health and Human Services, Statutes-at-a-Glance: Mandatory Reporters of Child Abuse and Neglect (2003) *http://childwelfare.gov/ systemwide/laws.policies/statutes/repproc.cfm.*

Childhelp USA® (www.childhelp.org) is a national organization that provides crisis assistance and other counseling and referral services. The Childhelp USA National Child Abuse Hotline is staffed 24 hours a day, 7 days a week, with professional crisis counselors who have access to a database of 55,000 emergency, social service, and support resources. All calls are anonymous. Childhelp USA can be contacted at (800) 4-A-CHILD, or (800) 422-4453.

RESOURCES

Quinn MJ, Tomita SK. *Elder abuse and neglect: causes, diagnosis, and intervention,* 2nd edition. — Springer Pub; 1997.

National Center on Elder Abuse: www.ncea.aoa.gov: The Center's mission is to promote understanding, knowledge sharing, and action on elder abuse, neglect and exploitation.

State Elder Abuse requirements can be found on the American Bar Association's web site at: www.abanet.ogr/aging/docs/MandatoryReportingProvisionsChart.pdf.

REFERENCES

1. Lachs MS, Pillemer K. Elder abuse. *Lancet.* 2004;364:1192–1263.

2. National Center on Elder Abuse: Administration on Aging: www.ncea.aoa.gov.

3. Lachs MS, et al. The mortality of elder mistreatment; *JAMA.* 1998;280(5):428–432.

4. Teaster PB. Sexual abuse of older adults: APS cases and outcomes. *Gerontologist.* 2004;44(6):788–786.

5. Mosqueda L, Dong X. Elder abuse and self-neglect: "I don't care anything about going to the doctor, to be honest . . . .". *JAMA.* 2011;306(5):532–540.

6. Mosqueda L, Dong X. Elder abuse and self-neglect: "I don't care anything about going to the doctor, to be honest . . . ."; JAMA. 2011;306(5):532–540.

7. Department of Health and Human Services, Administration for Children & Families. Chapter 2 Reports Child Maltreatment 2007. http://www.acf.hhs.gov/programs/cb/pubs/cm07/ chapter2.htm. Accessed November 2011.

8. Cincinnati Children's web site. Special Needs Resource Directory. http://www.cincinnati-childrens.org/patients/child/special-needs/family/abuse/. Accessed January 2012.

CHAPTER | SIXTEEN

Regulatory Compliance in Home Care Medicine

After reading this chapter you should be able to:

1. Identify key Centers for Medicare & Medicaid Services regulations related to physicians involved in home-based care

2. List examples of fraud and abuse and how to avoid them.

3. Describe compliance risk types and circumstances in home care medicine for which they apply

Physicians need to be aware of the importance of regulatory compliance. Many of the frequently encountered regulations come from the Centers for Medicare & Medicaid Services (CMS), following laws passed by Congress. Enforcement for CMS is performed by the Department of Health and Human Services Office of Inspector General (OIG). Many other parts of government have rules to which medical practices must adhere. In addition, contracts with payers and other organizations can add complexity to compliance.

This chapter is written by clinicians for clinicians and is NOT intended as a legal advice. Legal counsel related to compliance should be routine as part of program planning and implementation, especially when contracting between medical practices and other types of health care organizations.

Except when regulators or lawyers are at the door, education about regulatory compliance tends to bring yawns. Yet, when compliance problems are discovered, sleep deprivation is common. To make the topic maximally interesting to those not yet in trouble, a set of cases will be presented.

Practicing in the home setting or overseeing home health services has a unique set of circumstances and rules. Since many office- and hospital-based health care managers—and even health care attorneys—are unfamiliar with the home setting, physicians must become familiar with the issues that create risks to the provider or practice when caring for patients at home, directly or by overseeing other types of providers. Table 1 lists the assortment of risks associated with noncompliance, which can include loss of enrollment as a Medicare provider, loss of a medical license, fines, and jail. Table 2 provides a list of the various organizations that have rules that may apply to home medical practice.

TABLE 1 Compliance risk types and possible circumstances in home care medicine

Risk type	Example of possible circumstance	Possible penalty
Provision of unnecessary/ uncovered care	Home visits to a patient who could easily come to the office.	Denial of coverage, recovery of reimbursement, increased scrutiny of and delay in payment of future claims
Fraud and abuse	Signing a Medicare home care certification for a patient known to lack eligibility (e.g., not homebound) Accepting gifts or payments for referrals to a home health agency	Fine, loss of Medicare enrollment, jail
Malpractice	Failing to address medical follow-up needs (e.g., monitoring anti-coagulation, abnormal mammogram) for a patient unable to return to office because of physical immobility	Legal claim, filing with national malpractice databank
Unethical care—patient abandonment	Discontinuing home medical visits to patients without adequate arrangements for follow-up	Loss of medical license
Manslaughter	Withholding life-sustaining treatment for a patient (e.g., not calling 911) without documentation of an advance care plan	Jail
Breach of privacy	Well-intentioned sharing of medical information with a patients' family members against patient's expressed wishes, in order to organize home care or transition to other housing	Lawsuit, fines (if breach related to HIPAA)
Motor vehicle liability	Accident while traveling to/from patient home	Civil award not covered by insurance, loss of personal car insurance

TABLE 2 Organizations and agencies with regulatory authority over various aspects of home care medicine.

Federal

- ➤ Department of Health and Human Services (DHHS)

  - ➤ DHHS Centers for Medicare & Medicaid Services (CMS)

  - ➤ DHHS Office of Inspector General

  - ➤ DHHS Medicare Administrative Contractors (MACs – formerly "Carriers")

  - ➤ DHHS Office of Civil Rights (OCR -HIPAA Privacy and Security)

  - ➤ Drug Enforcement Administration (DEA)

  - ➤ Equal Employment Opportunity Commission (EEOC)

  - ➤ Internal Revenue Service (IRS)

  - ➤ Occupational Safety and Health Agency (OSHA)

State, County and Local

- ➤ Adult protection/vulnerable adults services (abuse and neglect)

- ➤ Boards of Medical Practice/Licensing

- ➤ Departments of Insurance/Insurance Commissioners

- ➤ Departments of Motor Vehicle

- ➤ Departments of Revenue/Taxation

- ➤ Hazardous waste regulators

- ➤ County and local regulations

- ➤ Offices of civil rights (discrimination)

Private (Civil) Parties

- ➤ Private (commercial) health insurers

- ➤ Contract Law

- ➤ Tort Law

IDENTIFYING RISKS

Every physician managing patients in the home understands, or quickly learns, how to balance the risks and benefits of having the patient stay at home versus going to an emergency department, hospital, or nursing home. Similarly, physicians must learn how to manage regulatory risks. It is often necessary to weigh the risk of non-compliant activities being discovered and the impact of the potential sanctions versus the costs of compliance. For example, multiple radiologists may review a mammogram to avoid missing a cancer and multiple office staff may examine a billing form to assure its accuracy before submission. At some point, the costs exceed the benefits.

The key CMS regulations of interest to physicians that relate to home-based care are:

➤ **Eligibility and coverage** of home health, hospice and durable medical equipment services. Physicians are at risk for inappropriately signing orders or certifications for these services.

➤ **Reimbursement** for physician activities related to home medical care. Billing for home visits, certification of home care episodes and care plan oversight have detailed rules substantially different from almost any other evaluation and management codes.

➤ **Limits on physicians' contractual relationships,** such as for service as a medical director for a home health agency. Significant penalties can apply if such relationships do not follow every aspect of regulations written for such contracting arrangements.

OTHER RISKS

Other risks to physicians and their practices arise in home medical care due to patient privacy requirements (e.g., when paper or electronic medical records leave the office or hospital), malpractice (especially when care is not coordinated or follow-up systems fail), or other liability (e.g., due to a car accident on the way to a home visit).

EXAMPLES OF POTENTIAL REGULATORY ISSUES ARE ILLUSTRATED BY THE FOLLOWING CASES:

Case 1. Expanding your practice

You are a partner in an emergency room medical practice. You are also a donor to and on the Board of a not-for-profit senior housing and nursing home campus.

The executive director asks if you would be willing to perform on-site medical visits to individuals in the assisted living and independent living buildings. The campus is willing to give you (at no cost) some office space for paperwork and calls (not to see patients). He suggests that this arrangement could lead to the campus' emergency medical care being preferentially referred to the hospital at which you work. He also thanks you for the occasional referral from your emergency room to the nursing home on the campus.

A. What tasks must be completed in order to meet regulatory or risk-reduction requirements before starting to see and bill Medicare for such visits?

➤ **Enroll in or update PECOS (Provider Enrollment, Chain and Ownership System)** – As of July 2010, physicians making referrals to home health agencies and durable medical equipment vendors are required to be enrolled in the CMS, web-based database, PECOS. Emergency room physicians would almost always be enrolled as part of their hospital practice, but an update would be necessary if additional locations of practice are added. There is a section specific to house calls, asking for the zip codes, county, or state in which such visits will occur. Another section asks for sites of care, including offices, hospitals or domiciliary homes (which includes assisted living buildings). This form asks for National Provider Identification (NPI) of each site. Most assisted living programs do not have such an NPI; if this is the case, the medical practice NPI should be substituted.

➤ **Notify medical malpractice carrier** – Most, if not all, medical malpractice carriers will include house calls and domiciliary visits in existing coverage. It is best to verify this with your carrier, however. Although there are no government regulations that require that providers have malpractice coverage for every type of service they provide, some employers, hospitals and health insurance programs have such an expectation. If such coverage is not included in existing policies, there are options to purchase such coverage separately.

➤ **Purchase appropriate equipment** – At least one Medicare carrier has a Local Carrier Decision (LCD) related to house calls that demands the quality of the house call service be comparable to an office visit. To achieve such a standard, basic diagnostic equipment and supplies must be carried by the physician. For a typical house call physician, this would include at least a blood pressure cuff, thermometer, oto/ophthalmoscope, stethoscope, oximeter, and reflex hammer. More advanced diagnostic technology, such as electrocardiography and point-of-service laboratory testing may be justified on clinical or economic grounds, but is not generally considered necessary under the "comparable quality" standard. For physicians in nonprimary care/urgent care practices, such as psychiatry, no diagnostic equipment may be necessary.

➤ **Develop consent forms** – Unlike the clinic or hospital setting, completion of consent forms is often part of the home care physician's activities. Three types of forms are required by regulations or contract.

1. **Billing consent/Assignment of Benefits** – Health insurers including CMS expect a signed consent allowing the provider to collect payments for services to the patient.

2. **Health Insurance Portability and Accountability Act (HIPAA)** – Patients must be offered a document describing their privacy rights under HIPAA. It is common, although not required, that patients sign a statement that they have received/refused receipt of this document. For more information on HIPAA go to http://www.cms.gov/hipaageninfo/ and see Appendix B.

3. **Release of information** – The house call provider usually needs records from prior or other clinicians. HIPAA requires that a release of information consent form be completed before medical records are transferred between nonconcurrent providers.

➤ **Notify auto insurance company** – Many automobile insurers require notification if an insured vehicle is used for on-the-job activities, rather than just for commuting.

B. What parts of the arrangement with the nursing home campus require careful legal review?

The cross-referral of patients to and from the emergency department represents normal medical practice, but the offer from the facility for use of free space by the physician in exchange for referrals may run afoul of anti-kickback and Stark regulations (http://www.starklaw.org).

Case 2. Spouse asks to be treated, too

You are visiting at home a 72-year-old man with a history of strokes that have led to dementia and immobility. He receives four hours per day of home aide care. His wife, aged 68 years, remains active and continues driving. During the visit to your patient, the wife tells you that she has symptoms, again, of a urinary tract infection. She asks if you would give her a prescription to refill her Ampicillin, which has worked in the past, since her clinic doctor has not returned her call from yesterday.

What could happen if you:

A. Write her the prescription, but do not enroll her as a patient in your practice, start a medical chart for her or bill for the service?

This, a generous and efficient option, has two potential consequences. First, state Boards of Medical Practice likely require maintenance of medical records as a condition of licensure. If a complaint was filed with the Board of Medical Practice, for example in the event that the wife had a serious reaction to the medication, sanctions could occur if medical records could not be produced in response to such a complaint (even if no other professional misconduct occurred). Example: NY state law § 6530 (28) and Minnesota statute 147.091 (o).

Second, it is possible that such a service provided to the wife of a patient could be considered an illegal gift, under section 1128A (a)(5) of the Social Security Act, enacted as part of Health Insurance Portability and Accountability Act of 1996 (HIPAA). That law prohibits individuals or entities from knowingly and willfully offering, paying, soliciting or receiving remuneration to induce referrals of items or services. Regulations have a limit of $10 individually, and no more than $50 in the aggregate annually per patient in value of items given to patients who receive Medicare-reimbursed services.

B. Enroll the wife as a patient in your practice, perform appropriate evaluation and management and bill Medicare for a house call to her, in addition to the husband.

The claim for such a house call could be denied on the basis that there was no reason she required a house call rather than an office visit. The Medicare carrier knows this is a house call based on both the Current Procedural Terminology (CPT) code used (99341-99350) and the Place of Service (POS) code required on the claim (12). If these CPT codes are used with any other POS code, the claim will be automatically rejected.

Although Medicare, nationally, has not defined the specifics of when a house call is justified, it does require that the provider document the reason the patient should be seen at home on each visit note. Several Medicare carriers have created policies, called Local Carrier Decisions (LCD), to clarify this issue across many parts of the country. Specifically, Medicare does NOT require that the patient be homebound according to the complex rules used for skilled home care benefits.

It is reasonable to consider (although not explicitly stated in regulations) that a house call could be justified to someone with caregiver responsibilities who lacks a reliable substitute to care for a disabled relative. In the case described, the husband has daily home aide services, so that the reason for visiting the wife is questionable. The medical record must document the medical necessity of the home visit made in lieu of an office or outpatient visit.

C. Enroll the wife as a patient in your practice, perform appropriate evaluation and management and bill Medicare using an office visit CPT code, in addition to billing for the house call for the husband.

Unfortunately, it is not compliant with rules to see a patient at home and bill it as if you saw the patient elsewhere (e.g., at your office).

D. Write a prescription for the antibiotics for the husband, to be available in case he develops an infection and tell the wife that no one can stop her from taking the medications herself.

This could be considered insurance fraud if the patient used health insurance to fill the prescription under such false pretenses. Risk of detection is minimal and risk to the physician is negligible, but the physician should consider the consequences of a police investigation should the wife have a serious reaction to the antibiotic and die.

Case 3. Uncle Louis and home health care benefit

You are the director of an urban academic geriatrics program. Your elderly aunt and uncle (Rita and Louis) live in a remote part of the same state on a farm. Although you keep in touch by phone, you haven't seen them in nine months. Aunt Rita reports that Louis has fallen down a few times. As he has for the past 10 years, he refuses to see a physician. They bought a cane, but he cannot manage using it and is not certain in which hand it should be held. They continue to go out for lunch a couple of times per week and to friends' homes once a week. The closest outpatient rehabilitation facility is 40 miles away and they prefer not to drive that far. The county hospital's home health agency does serve their community, however.

You agree to arrange for physical therapy through the home health agency. Given your need to maintain your clinical productivity, you also plan to bill for certification of home care and care plan oversight. What are the consequences of such a simple favor offered to a favorite aunt and uncle? All of the following are possible.

A. **The home health agency might not be paid for this admission.**

> Effective April 2011, federal law requires that the physician certifying Medicare-reimbursed skilled home care must have a recent face-to-face visit with the patient that documents the need for home care services and that the patient meets the homebound criteria (90 days prior or 30 days subsequent to the start of care).

> One consequence is that the home health agency might not be able to collect for the episode of care, unless Louis sees a physician for these falls within 30 days. That physician would have to sign paperwork for the home care agency.

B. **The home health agency might be cited for fraudulent billing** if it knowingly charges Medicare for a skilled home care episode for a patient who is not homebound. The frequency of out-of-home social activities is clearly inconsistent with the definition of homebound.

C. **You may be accused of fraudulently certifying an episode** of skilled home care by signing the certification form sent to you by the home health agency, which would state that you believe the patient is homebound or certify that you have seen the patient in the past 90 days.

D. **You may be accused of fraudulently billing Medicare** for certification of home care using billing code HCPCS G0180 as the patient was not eligible for skilled home care.

E. Even if you spend 30 minutes in a calendar month handling paperwork and phone calls regarding this episode of home care, **you may be accused of fraudulently billing Medicare for Care Plan Oversight** using HCPCS G0181 because that code requires that the physician has seen the patient in the prior six months.

F. Everything works out satisfactorily (and legally) when you persuade the home health agency to see your uncle at home using the outpatient rehabilitation billing codes.

> ➤ The Medicare outpatient rehabilitation benefit is not specific to any site, as it can be used in the clinic, outpatient areas of hospitals, nursing homes (when the patient is not on the Medicare skilled nursing facility benefit) and at home.

> ➤ The patient does not have to be homebound and the physician does not need to see the patient to order and oversee the care.

> ➤ The physician cannot bill for the certification of home care or care plan oversight.

> ➤ However, not all home health agencies have contracts with Medicare to provide outpatient rehabilitation. This is because the home health agency is paid per visit, typically less than the cost of travel, therapist salary and overhead.

Case 4. Managing your practice

Your house call practice is running smoothly with three doctors and six nurse practitioners. The practice has a managed care contract that pays a monthly capitation plus per visit fees and two home health medical directorships. In addition to visit fees for Medicare fee-for-service patients, you have been able to collect routinely for home care certification and care plan oversight, including for referrals to the agencies at which you offer medical direction. Your electronic medical record allows whoever takes night and weekend calls to enter care plan oversight notes. In addition, nurse practitioners manage home health agency phone calls during the day and carefully document these conversations. As a result, about half of the home care referrals lead to a care plan oversight charge at least once per episode of care. Are all these arrangements permissible?

A. Medicare Advantage plans and insurers for non-Medicare populations have begun to recognize the value of home-visiting physicians.

> ➤ A variety of payment arrangements are possible, including pure fee-for-service (at or above Medicare allowable rates), monthly case management or capitation fees, pay-for-performance (typically based on preventing hospitalization), risk sharing, and full risk contracting.

> ➤ For a practice of this size, a combination of monthly capitation and fee-for-service is a reasonable approach and permissible.

B. Referring patients to a home health agency with which you have a medical director contract can be legal and appropriate, if all relevant regulations and rules are followed. Specifically, the Medicare anti-kickback and self-referral (aka Stark) rules must have careful compliance.

> ➤ The contract with the agency must be in writing, must be for at least a year, must not have payments linked to numbers of referrals made

and must be for an amount consistent with **fair market value for physician time.**

➤ This can be determined through surveys by designated organizations of compensation for physicians in your specialty nationally and in your area.

➤ You will want to divide the proposed amount of compensation by the amount of time required to meet your contractual responsibilities to see if the compensation rate is consistent with the survey results.

➤ There is currently no limit to the total compensation that can be received as a medical director, as long as the hourly compensation is consistent with this determination of fair market value.

➤ Finally, you or a close relative cannot have an ownership interest in the agency (unless, for example, it is a publically traded corporation).

➤ It is also permitted for the home health agency medical director to perform the required face-to-face visit associated with an admission to skilled home care.

C. **Your description of tracking of time for billing of Care Plan Oversight to Medicare is very problematic. Only time spent by the physician who certified the episode of home care counts towards the 30 minutes per month required to bill this code.**

➤ Covering partners, office staff and other colleagues' time is irrelevant to this billing, although it is good malpractice avoidance and collaborative care to document all such communications in the medical record.

➤ Your nurse practitioners can use their time towards Care Plan Oversight if they are the primary clinician seeing the patient, but only one nurse practitioner can count such time per patient per episode of care.

RESOURCES

PECOS: https://www.cms.gov/MedicareProviderSupEnroll/04_InternetbasedPECOS.asp

HIPAA: http://www.cms.gov/hipaageninfo/

LCD for house calls: http://www.wpsmedicare.com/part_b/policy/active/local/l31613_phys081.shtml

Stark Law: http://www.law.cornell.edu/uscode/42/1395nn.html
http://www.starklaw.org

Miscellaneous issues: http://www.aahcp.org/displaycommon.cfm?an=1&subarticlenbr=151

CHAPTER | **SEVENTEEN**

Resources

State Departments on Aging

For the most up-to-date contact information and to find the closest agency on aging, as well as information on regional offices, consult the Eldercare Locator web site, *www.eldercare.gov* or call (800) 677-1116. The Eldercare Locator is maintained by the U.S. Department of Health and Human Services Administration on Aging.

Administration on Aging
One Massachusetts Avenue NW
Washington, DC 20201
Public Inquiries: (202) 619-0734
Asst Secretary for Aging: (202) 401-4634
Fax: (202) 357-3555
E-mail: aoainfo@aoa.hhs.gov
Eldercare Locator (to find local
Resources): (800) 677-1116
TDD: (800) 877-8339
www.aoa.gov

Alabama
Department of Senior Services
770 Washington Ave, RSA Plaza, Suite 570
Montgomery, AL 36130
877-425-2243
Fax: (334) 242-5594
E-mail: ageline@adss.alabama.gov
www.alabamaconnect.gov
http://www.adss.state.al.us

Alaska
Commission on Aging
Division of Senior Services

150 Third Street
PO Box 110693
Juneau, AK 99811-1398
(907) 465-4879
Fax: (907) 465-1398
www.alaskaaging.org

American Samoa
Territorial Administration on Aging
American Samoa Government
Pago Pago, American Samoa 96799
011 (684) 633-1251 or 633-1252
Fax: 011 (684) 633-2533
E-mail: taoa@americansomoa.gov
www.americansamoa.gov/department-type/
agency/administration-aging

Arizona
Aging and Adult Administration
Department of Economic Security
1789 W Jefferson St, #950A
Phoenix, AZ 85007
(602) 542-4446
Fax: (602) 542-6575
www.de.state.az.us/aaa

Arkansas

Division of Aging and Adult Services
Arkansas Dept of Human Services
700 Main Street
PO Box 1437, Slot S-530
Little Rock, AR 72203-1437
(501) 682-2441
Fax: (501) 682-8155
E-mail: aging.services@arkansas.gov
www.state.ar.us/dhs/aging

California

Department on Aging
1300 National Drive, Suite 200
Sacramento, CA 95834-1992
(916) 419-7500
Fax: (916) 928-2268
E-mail: webmaster@aging.ca.gov
TDD: (800) 735-2929
www.aging.state.ca.gov

Colorado

Division of Aging and Adult Services
1575 Sherman St, 10th Floor
Denver, CO 80203
(303) 866-2800
Fax: (303) 866-2696
TTY: (303) 866-2850
www.cdhs.state.co.us/oss/aas/

Connecticut

Aging Services Division
Department of Social Services
25 Sigourney Street, 10th Floor
Hartford, CT 06106
(860) 424-5274
Fax: (860) 424-5301
E-mail: agingservices.dss@ct.gov
TDD/TYY: (800)-842-4524
www.ctelderlyservices.state.ct.us

Delaware

Division of Services for Aging & Adults with
Physical Disabilities
Delaware Health and Social Services
1901 North DuPont Highway

New Castle, DE 19720
(800) 223-9074
Fax: (302) 255-4445
E-mail: DelawareADRC@state.de.us
TDD: (302) 391-3505 or (302) 424-7141
www.dsaapd.com

District of Columbia

Office on Aging
441 4th Street, NW, Suite 900 South
Washington, DC 20001
(202) 724-5622
Fax: (202) 724-4979
E-mail: dcoa@dc.gov
TTY: (202) 724-8925
www.dcoa.dc.gov

Florida

Department of Elder Affairs
4040 Esplanade Way
Tallahassee, FL 32399-7000
(850) 414-2000
Fax: (850) 414-2004
E-mail: *information@elderaffairs.org*
TDD: (850) 414-2001
http://elderaffairs.state.fl.us

Georgia

DHS Division of Aging Services
2 Peachtree St, NW, Suite 9-385
Atlanta, GA 30303-3142
(404) 657-5258
Fax: (404) 657-5285
E-mail: *dhrconstituentservices@dhr.state.ga.us*
http://aging.dhr.georgia.gov

Guam

Division of Senior Citizens
130 University Drive, Suite 8
University Castle Mall
Mangilao, Guam 96910
011 (671) 735-7011
Fax: 011 (671) 735-7316
TDD/TTY: 011 (671) 735-7315
www.dphss.guam.gov/about/senior_citizens.htm

Hawaii
Executive Office on Aging
No 1 Capitol District
250 South Hotel St, Suite 406
Honolulu, HI 96813-2831
(808) 586-0100
Fax: (808) 586-0185
E-mail: eoa@doh.hawaii.gov
www.hcoahawaii.org/

Idaho
Commission on Aging
341 W. Washington, 3rd Floor
Boise, ID 83720-0007
(208) 334-3833
Fax: (208) 334-3033
www.idahoaging.com

Illinois
Department on Aging
One Natural Resources Way, Suite 100
Springfield, IL 62702-1271
(217) 785-3356
Fax: (217) 785-4477
E-mail: aging.ilsenior@illinois.gov
TTY: (800) 206-1327
www.state.il.us/aging

Indiana
Division of Aging
402 W Washington St, PO Box 7083,
MS21 Room W-454
Indianapolis, IN 46204
(888) 673-0002
Fax: (317) 232-7867
http://www.in.gov/fssa/2329.htm

Iowa
Department on Aging
Jessie M. Parker Building
510 E. 12th Street, Suite 2
Des Moines, IA 50319-9025
(515) 725-3333
Fax: (515) 242-3300
E-mail: contactida@iowa.gov

TTY: (515) 725-3302
www.state.ia.us/elderaffairs

Kansas
Department on Aging
New England Bldg
503 S Kansas
Topeka, KS 66603-3404
(785) 296-4986
Fax: (785) 296-0256
E-mail: wwwmail@aging.ks.gov
TTY: (785) 291-3167
www.agingkansas.org

Kentucky
Department for Aging and Independent Living
Cabinet for Health and Family Services
Commonwealth of Kentucky
275 E Main St., 3E-E
Frankfort, KY 40621
(502) 564-6930
Fax: (502) 564-4595
TTY: (888) 642-1137
http://chs.ky.gov/dhss/das

Louisiana
Governor's Office of Elderly Affairs
525 Florida Street, 4th Floor
Baton Rouge, LA 70802
(225) 342-7100
Fax: (225) 342-7133
www.goea.louisiana.gov

Maine
Office of Elder Services
Department of Health and Human Services
11 State House Station
32 Blossom Lane
Augusta, ME 04333
(207) 287-9200
Fax: (207) 287-9229
TTY: (800) 606-0215
www.state.me.us/dhs/beas

Northern Mariana Islands
CNMI Office on Aging, DC & CA
PO Box 2178
Saipan, MP 96950
011 (671) 734-4361
Fax: 011 (670) 233-1327

Maryland
The Department of Aging
301 W Preston St, Suite 1007
Baltimore, MD 21201
(410) 767-1100
Fax: (410) 333-7943
E-mail: webmail@aoa.state.md.us
Relay service: (800) 201-7165
www.mdoa.state.md.us

Massachusetts
Executive Office of Elder Affairs
One Ashburton Place, 5th Floor
Boston, MA 02108
(617) 727-7750
Fax: (617) 727-9368
TTY: (800) 872-0166
www.800ageinfo.com

Michigan
Office of Services to the Aging
PO Box 30676
7109 West Saginaw Hwy
Lansing, MI 48909-8176
(517) 373-8230
Fax: (517) 373-4092
http://www.michigan.gov/miseniors

Minnesota
Board on Aging
Elmer L. Anderson Human Services Building
540 Cedar Street
St. Paul, MN 55155
(651) 431-2500 or
Fax: (651) 431-7453
TTY: (800) 627-3529
www.mnaging.org

Mississippi
Division of Aging and Adult Services
750 N State St
Jackson, MS 39202
(601) 359-4929
Fax: (601) 359-9664
E-mail: *aging@mdhs.ms.gov*
www.mdhs.state.ms.us/aas.html

Missouri
Department of Health and Senior Services
912 Wildwood
PO Box 570
Jefferson City, MO 65102
(573) 751-6400
Fax: (573) 751-6010
E-mail: info@ghss.mo.gov
www.dhss.mo.gov

Montana
Senior and Long Term Care Division
Department of Public Health & Human Services
PO Box 4210
2030 11th Avenue
Helena, MT 59620
(406) 444-4077
Fax: (406) 444-7743
http://www.dphhs.mt.gov/sltc

Nebraska
State Unit on Aging
Dept of Health & Human Services
Nebraska State Office Building
301 Centennial Mall South, 5th Floor
Lincoln, NE 68508
(402) 471-4623
Fax: (402) 471-4619
www.hhs.state.ne.us/ags/agsindex.htm

Nevada
Aging & Disability Services Division
Department of Health and Human Services
3416 Goni Rd, Bldg D, Suite 132
Carson City, NV 89706
(775) 687-4210

Fax: (775) 687-4264
http://aging.state.nv.us

New Hampshire
Bureau of Elderly and Adult Services
Division of Community Based Care Services
NH Division of Health and Human Services
129 Pleasant Street
Concord, NH 03301
(603) 271-4680
Fax: (603) 271-4643
TDD: (800) 735-2964
http://www.dhhs.nh.gov/dcbcs/beas/

New Jersey
Division of Aging and Community Services
Department of Health and Senior Services
PO Box 360
Trenton, NJ 08625-0360
(609) 292-7837
Fax: (609) 943-3343
www.state.nj.us/health/senior/sraffair.htm

New Mexico
Aging and Long-Term Services Department
Toney Anaya Building
2550 Cerrillos Road
Santa Fe, NM 87505
(505) 476-4799
Resource Center: (505) 476-4846
Fax: (505) 476-4836
www.nmaging.state.nm.us

New York
Office for the Aging
Two Empire State Plaza
Albany, NY 12223-1251
800-342-9871
Fax: (518) 474-1398
E-mail: nysofa@ofa.state.ny.us
www.aging.ny.gov

North Carolina
Division of Aging and Adult Services
Department of Health and Human Services

Taylor Hall, 693 Palmer Drive
Raleigh, NC 27603-2250
(919) 733-3983
Fax: (919) 733-0443
www.ncdhhs.gov/aging

North Dakota
Adults and Aging Services Division
Department of Human Services
1237 W. Divide Ave, Suite 6
Bismarck, ND 58501
(701) 328-4601
Fax: (701) 328-8744
E-mail: dhsaging@nd.gov
Relay TTY: (800) 366-6888
www.nd.gov/dhs/services/adultsaging/

Ohio
Department of Aging
50 W Broad St, 9th Fl
Columbus, OH 43215-3363
(614) 466-5500
Fax: (614) 466-5741
www.aging.ohio.gov/home/

Oklahoma
Aging Services Division
Department of Human Services
2401 N.W. 23rd Street, Suite 40
Oklahoma City, OK 73107
(405) 521-2281
Fax: (405) 521-2086
www.okdhs.org/divisionsoffices/visd/asd

Oregon
Senior and People with Disabilities
Department of Human Services
500 Summer St NE, E12
Salem, OR 97301-1073
(503) 945-5921
Fax: (503) 373-7823
E-mail: spd.web@state.or.us
TTY: (800) 282-8096
http://www.oregon.gov/DHS/spwpd/index.shtml

Pennsylvania
Department of Aging
555 Walnut St, 5th Fl
Harrisburg, PA 17101-1919
(717) 783-1550
Fax: (717) 783-6842
E-mail: aging@state.pa.us
www.aging.state.pa.us

Puerto Rico
Commonwealth of Puerto Rico
Puerto Rico Office of the Ombudsman
for the Elderly
PO Box 191179
San Juan, PR 00919-1179
(787) 721-6121
Fax: (787) 724-1152
www.oppea@gobierno.pr

Rhode Island
Department of Elderly Affairs
74 West Road
Hazard Building
Cranston, RI 02920
(401) 462-3000
Fax: (401) 462-0503
TTY: (410) 462-0740
www.dea.ri.gov

South Carolina
The Lieutenant Governor's Office on Aging
1301 Gervais Street, Suite 350
Columbia, SC 29201
(803) 734-9900
Fax: (803) 734-9886
E-mail: askus@aging.sc.gov
www.aging.sc.gov

South Dakota
Office of Adult Services and Aging
Richard F. Kneip Bldg
700 Governors Dr
Pierre, SD 57501
(605) 773-3656
Fax: (605) 773-4085
E-mail: ASA@state.sd.us
http://dss.sd.gov/elderlyservices

Tennessee
Commission on Aging and Disability
Andrew Jackson Bldg
500 Deaderick St, Suite 825
Nashville, TN 37243-0860
(615) 741-2056
Fax: (615) 741-3309
www.tn.gov/comaging/

Texas
Department of Aging and Disability Services
John H. Winters Human Services Complex
701 W 51st St
Austin, TX 78751
(512) 438-3011
E-mail: *mail@dads.state.tx.us*
www.dads.state.tx.us

Utah
Aging and Adult Services
195 North 1950 West
Salt Lake City, UT 841116
(801) 538-3910
Fax: (801) 538-4395
E-mail: *DAAS@utah.gov*
www.hsdaas.utah.gov

Vermont
Department of Disabilities, Aging &
Independent Living
103 South Main St
Weeks Building
Waterbury, VT 05671-1601
(802) 241-2401
Fax: (802) 241-2325
www.dail.vermont.gov

Virgin Islands
Senior Citizen Affairs
Department of Human Services
3011 Golden Rock Christiansted
St. Croix, VI 00820
(340) 773-2323
www.dhs.gov.vi/seniors/index.html

Virginia
Department for the Aging
1610 Forest Ave, Ste 100
Richmond, VA 23229
(804) 662-9333
Fax: (804) 662-9354
E-mail: *aging@vda.virginia.gov*
Nationwide Voice/TTY: (800) 552-3402
www.vda.virginia.gov

Washington
Aging and Disability Services Administration
Department of Social & Health Services
4550 10th Avenue SE
Lacey, WA 98503
(360) 725-2300
E-mail: *askdshs@dshs.wa.gov*
TTY: (877) 905-0454
www.adsa.dshs.wa.gov

West Virginia
Bureau of Senior Services
1900 Kanawha Blvd East
Charleston, WV 25305
(304) 558-3317
Fax: (304) 558-5609
www.wvseniorservices.gov

Wisconsin
Bureau of Aging and Disability Resources
Department of Health Services
1 W. Wilson St, Rm 450
PO Box 7851
Madison, WI 53707-7851
(608) 266-2536
Fax: (608) 267-3203
E-mail: DHFSDLTCAging@wisconsin.gov
TTY: (800) 701-1251
www.dhfs.state.wi.us/Aging

Wyoming
Aging Division Services
Department of Health
6101 Yellow Stone Rd, #259B
Cheyenne, WY 82002
(307) 777-7986 or (800) 442-2766
Fax: (307) 777-5340

E-mail: wyaging@health.wyo.gov
www.wyomingaging.org

National organizations/programs

Administration on Aging
One Massachusetts Avenue NW
Washington, DC 20201
(202) 619-0724
Fax: (202) 357-3555
E-mail: *AoAInfo@aoa.hhs.gov*
Eldercare Locator (local resources):
(800) 677-1116
www.aoa.gov

Agency for Healthcare Research and Quality (AHRQ)
AHRQ Health Care Innovations Exchange
540 Gaither Road
Rockville, MD 20850
(301) 427-1364
E-mail: info@innovations.ahrq.gov
www.innovations.ahrq.gov

Alzheimer's Disease and Related Disorders Association, Inc
225 N Michigan Ave, Ste 1700
Chicago, IL 60601-7633
(312) 335-8700 or (800) 272-3900
Fax: (866) 699-1246
TDD: (866) 403-3073
E-mail: *info@ALZ.org*
www.alz.org

American Academy of Home Care Physicians
PO Box 1037
Edgewood, MD 21040-0337
(410) 676-7966
Fax: (410) 676-7980
E-mail: *aahcp@comcast.net*
www.aahcp.org

American Academy of Hospice and Palliative Medicine
4700 W Lake Ave
Glenview, IL 60025-1485
(847) 375-4712

Fax: (877) 375-6433
E-mail: *info@aahpm.org*
www.aahpm.org

American Academy of Pediatrics National Center for Medical Home Implementation
141 Northwest Point Blvd
Elk Grove Village, IL 60007
(847) 434-4000
Fax: (847) 228-7035
E-mail: *medical_home@aap.org*
www.medicalhomeinfo.org

Association of Maternal and Child Health Programs
2030 M Street, NW, Suite 350
Washington DC 20036
(202) 775-0436
Fax: (202) 775-0061
E-mail: *info@amchp.org*
www.amchp.org

Centers for Medicare & Medicaid Services
7500 Security Blvd
Baltimore, MD 21244-1850
(877) 267-2323 or (410) 786-3000
TTY: (866) 226-1819

General: *www.cms.gov*
Home health agencies: *www.cms.gov/center/hha.asp*
Physicians: *www.cms.gov/center/physician.asp*

Childhelp USA
15757 N. 78th Street, Suite B
Scottsdale, AZ 85260
1-800-4-A-Child ((800) 422-4453)
www.childhelpusa.org

The Joint Commission
One Renaissance Blvd
Oakbrook Terrace, IL 60181
(630) 792-5000
Fax: (630) 792-5005
www.jointcommission.org

Family Caregiver Alliance
180 Montgomery Street, Suite 900
San Francisco, CA 94104 (415) 434-3388
www.caregiver.org

National Family Caregivers Association
10400 Connecticut Avenue, Suite 500
Kensington, MD 20895-3944
(800) 896-3659
www.nfcacares.org

CHAPTER | EIGHTEEN

Glossary of Home Care Terms

Activities of daily living (ADL): Self-care abilities related to personal care including bathing, dressing, eating, toileting, continence, transferring, and ambulating.

APS (adult protective services): These services protect vulnerable adults by investigating allegations of abuse, neglect, abandonment, and financial exploitation. Based on the outcome of an investigation, APS may offer legal or social protective services. An adult maintains the right to refuse protective services. The vulnerable adult or the legal representative must give written consent for protective services and may end the services at any time. APS conducts an investigation at no charge and without regard to the income of the alleged victim. Some protective services may be provided without cost.

Assessment: The process by which a physician or another health care professional evaluates a person's health status. Assessment is related to, but distinct from, diagnosis. It may involve the use of formal assessment instruments along with more informal interviews with the patient, the patient's family, and other caregivers, and with observation of the patient's behavior.

Assessment instruments: Specific procedures, tests, and scales used to measure and evaluate cognitive and self-care abilities, problems,

functional limitations, and other patient characteristics.

Attending physician: The physician designated by the patient or his or her representative who has the most significant role in the determinations and delivery of the individual's medical care.

Care plan oversight (CPO): Ongoing oversight of home care services after the physician has referred a patient to a home care agency and developed and/or approved the care plan. CPO can be done by the referring or another physician, nurse practitioner, or physician assistant identified by the referring physician. Oversight includes collaboration and communication between the referring physician and a variety of other health care professionals participating in the care of the patient.

Care transition: Care involved when a patient/client leaves one care setting (e.g., hospital, nursing home, assisted living facility, skilled nursing facility, primary care physician, home health provider, or specialist) and moves to another. It involves a set of actions designed to ensure the coordination of care as patients transfer between different locations.

Case management: Those activities necessary to determine the patient's needs, arrange for and coordinate the appropriate services, and monitor the effectiveness of services and reassess them as needed.

CHAP (*www.chapinc.org*): Community Health Accreditation Program of the National League for Nursing (NLN). CHAP was granted "deeming authority" by the Centers for Medicare & Medicaid Services (CMS) in 1992 for home health and in 1999, for hospice. This means that instead of state surveys, CHAP has regulatory authorization to survey agencies providing home health and hospice services to determine whether they meet the Medicare Conditions of Participation (COPs). In 2006, CMS granted CHAP full deeming authority for home medical equipment (HME).

Childhelp USA (www.childhelp.org): A national organization that provides crisis assistance and other counseling and referral services.

CLIA (Clinical Laboratory Improvement Amendments) (www.cms.gov/clia): The Centers for Medicare & Medicaid Services program that regulates all clinical laboratory testing in the United States. Some states (e.g., California) and professional societies (e.g., College of American Pathologists) have stricter guidelines.

CMN (Certificate of Medical Necessity): Forms required by Medicare to authorize certain categories of durable medical equipment.

CMS (Centers for Medicare & Medicaid Services) (www.cms.gov): The branch of the U.S. Department of Health and Human Services that issues rules and regulations for the Medicare and Medicaid programs.

Community-based Care Transitions Program (CCTP): The CCTP, mandated by section 3026 of the PPACA (Patient Protection and Affordable Care Act), provides funding to test models for improving care transitions for high-risk Medicare beneficiaries. The goals of the CCTP

are to improve transitions of beneficiaries from the inpatient hospital setting to other care settings, to improve quality of care, to reduce readmissions for high-risk beneficiaries, and to document measureable savings to the Medicare program (www.cms.gov/demoprojectsevalrpts/md/itemdetail.asp?itemid=CMS1239313).

Conditions of participation (www.cms.gov/CFCsAndCOPs/): The regulations under which a home health agency may be allowed to participate in Medicare and Medicaid programs.

Continuous improvement: A philosophy or attitude of looking for methods to improve the quality of products or services as an ongoing part of the administration of a health care delivery system.

Custodial care: Treatments or services, regardless of who recommends them or where they are provided, that could be given safely and reasonably by a person not medically skilled and are mainly to help the patient with activities of daily living.

Duplication of services: The same service being provided by two disciplines.

Durable medical equipment (DME): Defined by Medicare as equipment that can withstand repeated use, is primarily designed to serve a medical purpose, is generally not useful to a person in the absence of injury or illness, and is appropriate for use in the home. Examples of DME include oxygen concentrators, wheelchairs, walkers, hospital beds, and suction machines.

Enteral nutrition therapy: Therapy that addresses the nutritional needs of patients who are unable to take food orally. A feeding tube, passed through the nose, stomach, or small intestine, supplies the patient with calories and vital nutrients. Home enteral nutrition supplies and equipment are reimbursable under Medicare Part B for patients with Medicare-specified diagnoses.

The Federal Child Abuse Prevention and Treatment Act (CAPTA): CAPTA, as amended by the Keeping Children and Families Safe Act of 2003, defines child abuse and neglect.

CMS Form-485: Formerly required for home health certification and plan of care, now may be used or the HHA may submit any document that is signed and dated by the physician that contains all the data elements in the 485.

Fraud: Intentional deception or misrepresentation that an individual knows to be false and untrue.

Functional limitations: The limitations of performance and the impact of these limitations on the patient's lifestyle caused by chronic disease, either the broad effects of a single condition on many activities of daily life, or the independent effects of several conditions, each of which affects only a few activities.

HHS (U.S. Department of Health and Human Services): The department under which the Medicare and Medicaid programs are administered.

HIPAA (Health Insurance Portability and Accountability Act of 1996, P.L. 104-191) (www.cms.gov/hipaageninfo/): Title II of HIPAA concerns "Administrative Simplification." Title II is intended to improve the efficiency of the health care system by standardizing the electronic exchange of health care data and protecting the security and privacy of individuals' health care information.

High-technology home care: The application of technology at home to patients with acute, subacute, or chronic organ system diseases, dysfunction, or failure.

Home Based Primary Care (VA HBPC) (www.va.gov/GERIATRICS/Home_Based_Primary_Care.asp): Provides comprehensive, interdisciplinary, primary care in the homes of veterans with serious chronic disease and disability. HBPC targets frail, chronically ill veterans for whom routine clinic-based care is not effective. By providing coordinated care and the integration of diverse services, HBPC assists in improving the quality of life for these vulnerable individuals.

Hospital at Home: Hospital at Home is a care service delivery model that provides acute hospital-level care in the home as a substitute for care in a traditional acute hospital setting. It provides an intensity of care, including medical and nursing care, similar to that provided in the hospital, is appropriate to the severity of illness treated, and provides care that cannot be supplied by usual community-based home health care services. In the international literature, two general types of Hospital at Home models are described. "Substitutive" models usually divert patients from emergency department or ambulatory sites to the home. In this model, the patient is never admitted to the traditional hospital inpatient bed. In addition, "early discharge" models are described in which patients are initially admitted to the traditional acute hospital, and then later "transferred" to a Hospital at Home bed If the patient still requires acute hospital-level care.

Home health agency or organization (HHA): An organization that provides patients with skilled nursing and/or other therapeutic care in their homes, usually following the Medicare model of approved services (see home health care).

Home health aide: A trained individual who works under the supervision of a nurse or therapist, providing personal care and assistance with activities of daily living (ADL). Medicare requires that home health aides' training and competency evaluation must be completed before the aide renders care in the home.

Homebound: The patient has a condition, caused by an illness or injury, that restricts the ability of the patient to leave his or her home except with the assistance of another individual, or the aid of a supportive device (e.g., crutches, a cane, a wheelchair, or a walker), or the patient has a condition such that leaving his or her home is medically contraindicated.

Home care: Home care describes a vast array of services ranging from family members balancing the checkbook of a mildly demented parent, to nurse practitioners making post-natal visits to new parents, to skilled nurses, physical therapists, occupational therapists, speech therapists and social workers providing services to a recently discharged stroke patient, to physicians managing a ventilator-dependent patient in the patient's living room. It can also apply to vocational services, social services, homemaker services, and home health aide services to disabled, sick, or convalescent persons in the home. Services can range from high-technology care (e.g., administration of intravenous drugs) to relatively simple supportive care (e.g., provision of home-delivered meals).

Home health care: As defined under the Medicare Part A benefit, covers skilled, medically necessary care provided on an intermittent, part-time basis, by registered nurses, physical therapists, or speech therapists. If the patient qualifies for one or more of these "skilled" services, he or she is then eligible to receive services, if needed, from home health aides, dietitians, occupational therapists, and social workers.

Homemaker: A person paid to help in the home with personal care, light housekeeping, meal preparation, and shopping.

Instrumental activities of daily living (IADL): Activities that facilitate independence, such as the management of finances, use of the telephone, use of public transportation, meal planning and preparation, shopping, and taking medications appropriately.

Intermediary: The organization handling claims from hospitals, nursing homes, home health agencies, and other health care providers under federal or state health coverage programs.

Intermittent: A qualifying criterion for Medicare home health services, meaning that continuous 24-hour/day nursing services will not be covered, but only those services "either provided or needed on fewer than 7 days each week or less than 8 hours each day and 28 or fewer hours each week for periods of 21 days or less with extensions in exceptional circumstances when the need for additional care is finite and predictable." Most Medicare home health patients do not require such intensive services.

The Joint Commission (www.jointcommission.org) (formerly JCAHO: Joint Commission on Accreditation of Healthcare Organizations): An independent, not-for-profit organization, The Joint Commission accredits and certifies more than 19,000 health care organizations and programs in the United States including hospitals, ambulatory health care, behavioral health care, nursing home care, as well as home health care and durable medical equipment organizations.

Management and evaluation of the care plan: Skilled nursing visits for management and evaluation of the patient's care plan under the Medicare home health benefit are considered "reasonable and necessary where underlying conditions or complications require that only a registered nurse can ensure that essential nonskilled care is achieving its purpose. For skilled nursing care to be reasonable and necessary for management and evaluation of the patient's plan of care, the complexity of the necessary unskilled services that are a necessary part of the medical treatment must require the involvement of licensed nurses to promote the patient's recovery and medical safety in view of the patient's overall condition".

Medicaid (Title XIX): A state/federal program designed to provide medical benefits to indigent persons of all ages.

Medically necessary care (under Medicare): "To be considered reasonable and necessary, services must be consistent with the nature and severity of the patient's illness or injury, his or her particular medical needs, and the accepted standards of medical and nursing practice, without regard as to whether the illness or injury is acute, chronic, terminal, or expected to last a long time."

Medical necessity: Services required and medically appropriate for the treatment of an illness or injury. Such services must be consistent with recognized standards of care.

Medical social services: Social services in home care are directly related to the treatment of the patient's medical condition. Medicare allows two to three visits for family intervention directly related to the patient's health and safety.

Medicare: Public Law 89-97, which provides hospital and physician benefits for eligible persons (aged 65 years or older, permanently disabled after 24 consecutive months of disability, or those with chronic renal disease who require hemodialysis or kidney transplant after a three-month waiting period). Medicare Part A provides hospital and home health benefits; Medicare Part B provides benefits for professional services, durable medical equipment (DME), and supplies.

Medicare-certified: A home health agency or organization that is found by the Centers for Medicare & Medicaid Services (CMS) to meet Medicare's Conditions of Participation, is certified by CMS, and is thus allowed to participate in the Medicare program.

Medicare criteria for skilled services: "To be considered a skilled service, the service must be so inherently complex that it can be safely and effectively performed only by, or under the supervision of, professional or technical personnel."

Medicare's OASIS: See OASIS.

Mini-Mental State Examination (MMSE): A simple screening test to detect dementia; it assesses a range of cognitive abilities, such as memory, calculations, language, and spatial ability.

The National Center on Elder Abuse (NCEA) (*www.ncea.aoa.gov*): Useful national resource for elder rights, law enforcement and legal professionals, public policy leaders, researchers, and the public administered under the auspices of the National Association of State Units on Aging. Its Web site has links to state adult protective services web sites and other useful information on elder abuse.

NAHC National Association for Home Care and Hospice (www.nahc.org): A membership organization of home health agencies, hospices and home care aide organizations

NCQA (National Committee for Quality Assurance) (www.ncqa.org): Founded in 1979, the NCQA performs external review of quality assurance programs in prepaid health plans.

NLN (CHAP): National League for Nursing's Community Health Accreditation Program (see under CHAP above).

Nutritional services: The assessment, planning, and recommendations for a patient's nutritional needs by a dietitian.

OASIS (Outcome and Assessment Information Set) (www.cms.gov/ HomeHealthQualityInits/06_OASISC.asp): The instrument/data collection tool used to collect and report performance data by home health agencies. Since 1999, CMS has required Medicare-certified home health agencies to collect and transmit OASIS data for all adult patients whose care is reimbursed by Medicare and Medicaid with the exception of patients receiving pre- or postnatal services only. OASIS data are used for multiple purposes including calculating several types of quality reports which are provided to home health agencies to help guide quality and performance improvement efforts. Beginning in January 2010 the latest version OASIS-C includes data items supporting measurement of rates for use of specific evidence-based care processes. From a national policy perspective, CMS anticipates that these process measures will promote the use of best practices across the home health industry. Selected OASIS items are also used to define case-mix payments for the 60-day episode.

Occupational therapy services: Assist the patient to attain the maximum level of physical motor skills, sensory testing, adaptive or assistive devices, activities of daily living, and specialized upper extremity/hand therapies. While occupational therapy does not, in itself, constitute a basis for entitlement to Medicare reimbursement, a beneficiary of home health services (i.e., skilled nursing care, physical, and/or speech therapy) is also covered for occupational therapy.

Outcomes Based Quality Improvement (OBQI): OBQI Reports include 37 risk-adjusted outcome measures from OASIS-C. These reports allow home health agencies to proceed into the second phase of OBQI, called outcome enhancement. It is the outcome enhancement activities that allow an agency to focus its quality (or performance) improvement activities on select target outcomes, to investigate the care processes that contributed to these outcomes, and to make changes in clinical actions that will lead to improved patient outcomes. If the agency carefully implements the steps in this process, this change in patient outcomes is expected to be evident when the next report is accessed. (www .cms.gov/HomeHealthQualityInits/Downloads/ HHQIOBQIManual.pdf)

PACE (Program of All Inclusive Care for the Elderly) (www.cms.gov/pace): PACE is an optional benefit under both Medicare and Medicaid in which dually eligible persons who are frail enough to meet state standards for nursing home care are offered an alternative to institutionalization. Under PACE, they are offered comprehensive medical and social services through adult day centers and home and/or inpatient facilities. PACE is available only in states that have chosen to offer it under Medicaid.

Parenteral nutrition therapy: Therapy to assist patients unable to digest food by the gastrointestinal tract. A catheter, usually centrally placed and attached to an infusion pump, supplies nutrients to the patient's bloodstream. Supplies and equipment are reimbursable under Medicare Part B for patients with Medicare-specified diagnoses.

Patient Protection and Affordable Care Act (PPACA): Federal health care reform legislation enacted 2010.

PECOS (Provider Enrollment, Chain and Ownership System): As of July 2010, physicians making referrals to home health agencies and durable medical equipment vendors are required to be enrolled in the CMS, web-based database, PECOS.

Personal care: Assistance with activities of daily living, including bathing, toileting, dressing, grooming, transferring and feeding.

Physical therapy services: The treatment of neuromuscular and musculoskeletal dysfunctions through the application of physical agents (heat, cold, ultrasound, etc.) and neuromuscular procedures to alleviate pain, prevent disability, and rehabilitate function after disease or trauma. Services are based on patient need and should have a restorative function. This usually means that the patient has a fair or good rehabilitation potential. The physical therapy documentation must show progress toward established goals.

Primary family caregiver or care partner: Relative or significant other who assumes many of the tasks involved in caring for a home care patient that the patient is unable to perform.

Private-duty nursing: Nursing, chore service, housekeeping, and other types of patient care administered in a hospital, in a nursing home, or by a home health agency. Private-duty nursing is covered by some private-pay insurers or is self-pay.

Psychiatric nursing: The nurse must meet specific credentialing and training requirements to perform home health psychiatric nursing. Psychiatric nurses specialize in caring for home care patients with mental disorders but should also be able to perform other aspects of home health such as wound care.

Quality control: A management process where performance is measured against expectations and corrective actions are taken as needed.

Recertification: The attending physician certifies that the beneficiary requires continued skilled services after the expiration date of the initial certification, and then periodically thereafter.

Respiratory care services: Required by patients who suffer from a variety of chronic pulmonary or heart related problems. Home respiratory care treatment (oxygen therapy, intermittent positive-pressure breathing [IPPB] therapy, etc.) is covered under Medicare Part B, based on criteria of medical necessity.

Respite care: Services provided on a short-term basis to individuals unable to care for themselves. Respite care provides a relief (respite) for those persons normally providing care to the individual, allowing these caregivers time off to attend to their own needs or the needs of other family members.

Skilled nursing services: Occurs when a registered nurse uses knowledge as a professional nurse to execute skills, render judgments, and evaluate process and outcomes. The skills allowed in home health are assessment and observation, teaching and training, direct procedures, and management and evaluation of the care plan.

Speech therapy services: Provided by a speech and language therapist as part of the home rehabilitation program for patients with cerebrovascular accidents, tracheostomies, laryngectomies, and various neuromuscular diseases.

Telehealth: Technology that allows remote monitoring of a patient. It can include transmitting patient data, such as weight, vital signs, and blood sugar levels, to two-way video communication and listening devices (e.g., telestethoscopes) in order to conduct virtual health care visits.

AMA Caregiver Self-Assessment Questionnaire

Caregiver self-assessment questionnaire
How are YOU?

Caregivers are often so concerned with caring for their relative's needs that they lose sight of their own well-being. Please take just a moment to answer the following questions. Once you have answered the questions, turn the page to do a self-evaluation.

During the past week or so, I have ...

1. Had trouble keeping my mind on what I was doing .... ☐ Yes ☐ No

2. Felt that I couldn't leave my relative alone .... ☐ Yes ☐ No

3. Had difficulty making decisions .... ☐ Yes ☐ No

4. Felt completely overwhelmed ...... ☐ Yes ☐ No

5. Felt useful and needed .... ☐ Yes ☐ No

6. Felt lonely .... ☐ Yes ☐ No

7. Been upset that my relative has changed so much from his/her former self .... ☐ Yes ☐ No

8. Felt a loss of privacy and/or personal time .... ☐ Yes ☐ No

9. Been edgy or irritable .... ☐ Yes ☐ No

10. Had sleep disturbed because of caring for my relative .... ☐ Yes ☐ No

11. Had a crying spell(s) .... ☐ Yes ☐ No

12. Felt strained between work and family responsibilities .... ☐ Yes ☐ No

13. Had back pain .... ☐ Yes ☐ No

14. Felt ill *(headaches, stomach problems or common cold)* .... ☐ Yes ☐ No

15. Been satisfied with the support my family has given me .... ☐ Yes ☐ No

16. Found my relative's living situation to be inconvenient or a barrier to care .... ☐ Yes ☐ No

17. On a scale of 1 to 10, with 1 being "not stressful" to 10 being "extremely stressful," please rate your current level of stress.

_____

18. On a scale of 1 to 10, with 1 being "very healthy" to 10 being "very ill," please rate your current health compared to what it was this time last year. _____

Comments:
(Please feel free to comment or provide feedback.)

_____

_____

_____

_____

_____

_____

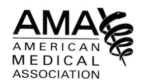

AMERICAN MEDICAL ASSOCIATION

Self-evaluation

To determine the score:

1. Reverse score questions 5 and 15.
   (For example, a "No" response should be counted as "Yes" and a "Yes" response should be counted as "No.")
2. Total the number of "yes" responses.

To interpret the score

Chances are that you are experiencing a high degree of distress:

- If you answered "Yes" to either or both questions 4 and 11; or
- If your total "Yes" score = 10 or more; or
- If your score on question 17 is 6 or higher; or
- If your score on question 18 is 6 or higher

Next steps

- Consider seeing a doctor for a check-up for yourself
- Consider having some relief from caregiving (Discuss with the doctor or a social worker the resources available in your community.)
- Consider joining a support group

Valuable resources for caregivers

Eldercare Locator
(a national directory of community services)
(800) 677-1116
www.eldercare.gov

Family Caregiver Alliance
(415) 434-3388
www.caregiver.org

Medicare Hotline
(800) 633-4227
www.medicare.gov

National Alliance for Caregiving
(301) 718-8444
www.caregiving.org

National Family Caregivers Association
(800) 896-3650
www.nfcacares.org

National Information Center for Children and Youth with Disabilities
(800) 695-0285
www.nichcy.org

Local resources and contacts:

Additional Information on HIPAA, OASIS and OBQI Regulations

THE HEALTH INSURANCE PORTABILITY AND ACCOUNTABILITY ACT (HIPAA) PRIVACY RULE

"HIPAA" refers to the federal "Health Insurance Portability and Accountability Act of 1996," P.L. 104-191. Title II of HIPAA concerns "Administrative Simplification." Title II is intended to improve the efficiency of the health care system by standardizing the electronic exchange of health care data and protecting the security and privacy of individuals' health care information. The HIPAA privacy rule is a lengthy and detailed regulation providing extensive and comprehensive federal protection for the privacy of health information that affects all health care providers, including home health agencies (HHAs) and hospices. Compliance with HIPAA involves all aspects of an HHA's or hospice's operation and will be a continuing cost to those providers.[1]

Who is covered? HIPAA covers health plans, health care clearinghouses, and those health care providers who transmit any health information in electronic form in connection with a HIPAA-covered transaction. HIPAA-covered transactions are:

➤ Health claims or equivalent encounter information

➤ Health claims attachments

➤ Enrollment and disenrollment in a health plan

➤ Eligibility for a health plan

➤ Health care payment and remittance advice

➤ Health plan payments

➤ First report of injury

➤ Health claims status

➤ Referral certification and authorization

Who is a "health care provider"? According to HIPAA, a "health care provider" is a provider of services for purposes of Medicare, a provider of medical or health services for purposes of Medicare, and "any other person or organization who furnishes, bills, or is paid for health care in the normal course of business." "Health care" includes, but is not limited to, "preventive, diagnostic, therapeutic, rehabilitative, maintenance, or palliative care, and counseling, services, assessment, or procedure with respect to the physical or mental condition, or functional status, of an individual or that affects the structure or function of the body; and sale or dispensing of a drug, device, equipment, or other item in accordance with a prescription."

Penalties for noncompliance Since April 14, 2003, virtually all home health providers and hospices must comply with the privacy rule's requirements. If not, HIPAA provides for civil penalties of $100 per incident, up to $25,000 per person, per year, per standard. It also permits criminal penalties ranging up to $250,000 and up to 10 years in prison. Concerns about HIPAA should not compromise the quality of home care. Compliance with the HIPAA regulations does not preclude communications between health care providers involved in the patient's care as long as the provider knows with whom he or she is communicating, the provider has reasonable confidence that the communication is secure so that the patient's medical information is kept private, and the provider keeps a record of communications. A general blanket waiver should be included in the initial enrollment papers signed by patients and families that authorizes providers to share medical information as needed with other medical providers involved in the patient's care. A copy and information concerning the privacy rule and guidance may be found at *www.hhs.gov/ocr/hipaa.*

OUTCOME AND ASSESSMENT INFORMATION SET (OASIS)

All HHAs that participate with Medicare are required to use a specific clinical assessment tool called the Outcome and Assessment Information Set (OASIS), and for all Medicare patients, the agencies must submit the OASIS data to a central database for use in quality improvement. The 89-item OASIS assessment is oriented to functionality and symptom improvement, is designed to evaluate the key endpoints that are important in home care, and has been extensively tested for validity. A full OASIS must be completed at entry to home care and at discharge. The requirements for interval assessments are being reworked. Although OASIS is lengthy, when the OASIS items are incorporated as part of the patient assessment instrument (replacing other items, rather than "added on") and performed by a trained and experienced provider, OASIS does not add time to the assessment process. OASIS is now used for dual purposes: quality improvement (the original purpose when OASIS was designed) and payment (a later use of OASIS, added when the Prospective Payment System [PPS] was developed). About one quarter of the OASIS items are used for payment to determine assignment of the patient into one of the 80 PPS categories

OUTCOMES BASED QUALITY IMPROVEMENT (OBQI)

Prior to the PPS, 10 years of research was conducted on quality improvement in Medicare home health, focusing on 41 outcomes and leading to the development of the CMS Outcomes Based Quality Improvement (OBQI) initiative. In two concurrent major demonstrations, altogether involving nearly 250,000 patients in 19 states and 73 agencies, demonstration (intervention) agencies were given feedback on their outcomes, adjusted for differences in case-mix.[2] The agencies were carefully trained in how to read the OBQI reports and how to use them for quality improvement. They received no other intervention. Comparison patients received care from other agencies similar in size and geography. Targeted outcomes improved significantly in the intervention agencies, while outcomes that were not targeted for improvement showed no change. Importantly, hospitalization was one of the targeted outcomes, and a 25% annual reduction in hospitalization was documented for patients cared for by agencies that were in the intervention group. Subsequently, state-level replications of these studies have demonstrated similar results.

The OBQI program is now an ongoing national initiative that is required for all agencies. As part of this effort, the content (items) and the application of OASIS (frequency of assessment, number of items) is being revised and updated on a continuing basis. Additionally, 11 OASIS items are now being used for posting public reports on the quality of care provided by home health agencies. These reports appear on the CMS Web site. The OASIS and OBQI efforts are a watershed event in home health care. This is the first time there have been reliable national-level data about these patients and about the impact of services rendered through home care. Home care has suffered from being a "black box" and the lack of measures that could be used for accountability. This is also particularly important now that the PPS creates an incentive for agencies to provide fewer services. From a physician perspective, OASIS and OBQI are likely "invisible" since OASIS data are not sent to physicians, and physicians normally do not need to see the OASIS. Review of OASIS is also not required for any physician activity, including billing for care certification or care plan oversight. The impact of OBQI on the improvement of quality is enormously important to physicians and their patients.

REFERENCES

1. Adapted from: *The Remington Report HIPAA Privacy Compliance Resource Manual* and published with permission of the author and copyright owner, John C. Gilliland II, Attorney at Law, Gilliland & Caudill LLP, 6650 Telecom Drive, Suite 100, Indianapolis, Indiana 46278, *jcg@gilliland.com*. *Information on the HIPAA Privacy Compliance Resource Manual* can be obtained by contacting Mr. Gilliland directly or from his firm's Web site (*www.gilliland.com*).

2. Shaughnessy PW, Hittle DF, Crisler KS, Powell MC, Richard AA, Kramer AM, et al. Improving patient outcomes of home health care: findings from two demonstrations of outcome-based quality improvement. *J Am Geriatr Soc.* 2002;50:1354-1364.

Continuing Medical Education

CME QUESTIONS FOR MEDICAL MANAGEMENT OF THE HOME CARE PATIENT

1. Reasons why house calls are on the rise include all the following except:
   a. Demographics (aging of society)
   b. Portable technology that allows sophisticated care in the home
   c. Home health agencies supporting house call programs by paying for referrals
   d. CMS (Centers for Medicare & Medicaid Services) increasing payments for house calls
   e. Legislation incentivizing house calls, such as the Independence at Home Act, and penalizing hospitals for readmissions

2. The largest payer of skilled home health care is:
   a. Private insurance
   b. Medicare
   c. Medicaid
   d. Veterans Administration
   e. Patient or family out-of-pocket

3. The largest payer of nonskilled (custodial care) is:
   a. Private insurance
   b. Medicare
   c. Medicaid
   d. Veterans Administration
   e. Patient or family out-of-pocket

4. Advantages of making a house call include:
   a. Identification of home health care needs
   b. Determining the needs of the caregivers
   c. Evaluating the patient's environment
   d. A and c only
   e. All the above

5. Patient assessments that can be done in the home include:
   a. ADLs/IADLs
   b. Mental status examination
   c. Environmental assessment
   d. B and c only
   e. All the above

6. True/False: The value of family caregiver services in the United States is estimated to be almost double what is actually spent on home care and nursing home services combined.

7. Medicare-covered home health care services include all the following except:
   a. Nursing
   b. Physical therapy
   c. Occupational therapy
   d. Respite
   e. Social work

8. Factors that should be considered in choosing a Medicare-certified home health agency include all the following except:
   a. The agency's accreditations
   b. Results of state and federal surveys such as Home Health Compare
   c. The agency's willingness to provide phlebotomy services as the sole skilled need
   d. Whether the agency employs most of the providers or uses subcontractors
   e. How the agency covers after hours and weekends

9. Under the Patient Protection and Affordable Care Act, to authorize home health care a physician (or a nurse practitioner or a physician assistant working for or in collaboration with a physician) must have a face-to-face encounter with the patient and document the need for home health care:
   a. 30 days before or 30 days after start of care
   b. 60 days before or 60 days after start of care
   c. 90 days before or 90 days after start of care
   d. 90 days before or 30 days after start of care
   e. A face-to-face encounter is not required as long as the physician knows the patient

10. Family caregivers to the aged and disabled provide what percentage of care in the community?
    a. 20%
    b. 40%
    c. 60%

d. 80%

e. 100%

11. Topics of special importance to pediatric home care patients include:

a. Optimal nutrition and feeding

b. Modification of technology support for optimal functioning

c. Education and socialization needs

d. Family/marital stress due to parenting a child with special needs

e. All the above

12. Marge is an 82-year-old woman with mild dementia who was recently hospitalized with her first episode of congestive heart failure. After her hospitalization she is having some difficulty walking and her doctor orders a walker and a home health nurse to teach Marge about congestive heart failure and physical therapy to improve her gait. The patient and family are agreeable to home health care but desire that Marge continue going to adult day care three times per week and attending church once a week. Which of the following is correct?

a. The patient does not qualify as she is able to go out to day care and attend church services

b. The patient can get home health care if the patient stops going to day care and attending church while she is receiving home health care

c. The patient can get home health care and the patient can go to day care and attend church

d. The patient can get home health and the patient can go to church but not to day care

e. The patient can get home health and the patient can go to day care but not to church

13. Medicare will pay physicians for all of the following except:

a. Certifying a patient for home health care

b. Recertifying a patient for home health care

c. Spending 30 minutes in a calendar month talking to home health personnel

d. Spending 30 minutes in a calendar month speaking to nurses at assisted living facilities

e. Making a house call

14. The form to certify and recertify Medicare home health patients includes all the following information except:

a. Patient demographic information

b. Medicare number and supplemental insurance information

c. Diagnoses

d. Medications

e. Prognosis

15. Home health agencies are required to provide the following services except:

a. Nursing

b. Pharmacy

c. Physical therapy

d. Occupational therapy

e. Social workers

16. Factors to consider when choosing a home health agency include:

a. The agency's accreditation (The Joint Commission or Community Health Accreditation Program)

b. What insurance the agency accepts

c. Results on Home Health Compare

d. A and c only

e. All the above

17. Medicare Home Health covers all the following services except:

a. Nursing

b. Physical, occupational and speech therapy

c. Home health aide services

d. Homemaker services

e. Social worker services

18. Services that can be provided by local Area Agencies on Aging can include all the following except:

a. Meals on Wheels

b. Homemaker services

c. Medicare-certified home health

d. Pharmaceutical assistance

e. Utility assistance

19. Which of the following may be involved in case management services?

    a. A patient needs assessment

    b. Arranging for and coordinating appropriate services

    c. Monitoring effectiveness of services

    d. A and b only

    e. All the above

20. Which of the following services cannot be provided in the home?

    a. Blood transfusions

    b. Intravenous antibiotics

    c. PICC (peripherally inserted central catheter) line insertion

    d. Ventilator management

    e. All the above can be provided in the home

21. Which of the following technology services cannot be provided in the home?

    a. Point-of-care blood tests such as international normalized ratio (INR), chemistries

    b. Arterial blood test

    c. Electrocardiogram

    d. Ultrasound

    e. All the above technologies can be done in the home

22. Which of the following is true concerning the Medicare hospice benefit?

    a. A patient can initiate hospice without a doctor's order

    b. The majority of patients on hospice live more than one month

    c. Medicare patients are allowed up to six months of hospice care

    d. The patient must have a "Do Not Attempt Resuscitation" order to sign up for hospice

    e. When the patient dies no further services are provided to the family

23. The hospice benefit pays for all the following except:

    a. Nursing services

    b. Home health aide, social worker and chaplain services

    c. Funeral costs

    d. Medications for comfort

    e. Durable medical equipment

24. Which of the following is true?

    a. It is allowable to accept compensation from a home health agency for a referral as long as the payment is "reasonable and customary"

    b. It is allowable for a durable medical equipment company to fill out a Certificate of Medical Necessity for a doctor to review as they are more knowledgeable about the equipment.

    c. Physicians have been criminally prosecuted for accepting fees from home health agencies for referrals

    d. It is allowable to accept compensation from a durable medical equipment company for the time taken to fill out a Certificate of Medical Necessity as long as the payment is "reasonable and customary"

    e. Home health agencies can offer hospitals free services such as nurses for discharge planning in exchange for referrals

25. Under Medicare home health conditions of participation a patient has the right to:

    a. Know how much care will cost, how payments will be handled, and whether the patient is responsible for any of those payments

    b. Be advised of potential conflicts of interest that physicians may have

    c. Participate actively in the design of a care plan, and help update it as needs change.

    d. Be advised of the availability of the toll-free home health agency hotline(s) (telephone number varies by state)

    e. All the above

    f. None of the above

26. Which of the following is not true about elder abuse?

    a. The estimated frequency of elder abuse is 2% to 10%

    b. The typical abuser is a "burned out" caregiver

c. Less than 10% of abuse is reported to authorities

d. Once reported, the majority of abused elders agree to press charges

e. Mandatory reporting of elder abuse is required in a majority of states

27. The most common form of elder abuse is:

a. Self-neglect

b. Active neglect

c. Physical abuse

d. Emotional abuse

e. Financial abuse

28. You are visiting at home a 72-year-old man with a history of strokes, which have led to dementia and immobility. He receives four hours per day of homemaker care. His wife, aged 68 years, remains active and continues driving. During the visit to your patient, the wife tells you that she has symptoms, again, of a urinary tract infection. She asks if you would give her a prescription for Ampicillin, which has worked in the past, since her clinic doctor has not returned her call from yesterday. What answer below would comply with federal regulations?

a. Write her the prescription, but do not enroll her as a patient in your practice, start a medical chart for her or bill for the service

b. Enroll the wife as a patient in your practice, perform appropriate evaluation and management and bill Medicare for a house call to her, in addition to the husband.

c. Enroll the wife as a patient in your practice, perform appropriate evaluation and management and billed Medicare using an office visit Current Procedural Terminology (CPT) code, in addition to billing for the house call for the husband.

d. Write a prescription for the antibiotics for the husband, to be available in case he develops an infection and tell the wife that no one can stop her from taking the medications herself.

e. None of the above.

29. Which of the following is true concerning the Veterans Administration's Home Based Primary Care (HBPC) Program?

a. Veterans cannot receive both the HBPC program and Medicare-covered home health care

b. To receive the HBPC program the veteran and caregiver must be willing to accept HBPC as their primary care provider and coordinator of care

c. Veterans must meet the government's definition of "homebound" to receive the HBPC program

d. Any veteran in the continental United States who medically qualifies can receive the HBPC program

e. Veterans on the VA's HBPC program have better health outcomes but the costs are higher than those for similar VA patients not on the program

30. True/False: The VA Home Based Primary Care (HBPC) program has high patient satisfaction at only slight increased cost over standard care.

31. One of the goals of focusing on care transitions is to reduce preventable readmissions. Medicare claims data from 2003-2004 regarding hospital discharges indicate what percentage of patients are readmitted within 30 days of discharge?

a. 5%

b. 10%

c. 15%

d. 20%

e. 25%

32. Elements that should be a part of quality transitional care from hospital to home include:

a. The site sending the patient maintains responsibility for the patient until the receiving site assumes care

b. The patient participates in decisions and patient information arrives with or prior to the patient

c. Medication reconciliation is performed by both the sending and the receiving entities

d. A and c only

e. All the above

33. The percentage of new Medicare-reimbursed home care episodes following hospital inpatient care is:

a. 25%

b. 33%

c. 50%

d. 66%

e. 75%

34. For every patient over age 65 years residing in a nursing home, how many similarly impaired patients are residing in their own homes?

a. 1

b. 2

c. 3

d. 4

e. 5

35. According to the June 2011 Medicare Payment Advisory Commission (MEDPAC) report, the costliest 10% of Medicare health care users consumed what percentage of the total Medicare costs?

a. 27%

b. 37%

c. 47%

d. 57%

e. 67%

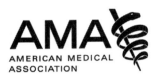

CME ACTIVITY EVALUATION FORM
Medical Management of the Home Care Patient: Guidelines for Physicians
4th Edition

As a result of participating in this activity, I am able to:

Describe the scope of home care and the populations that use it.	**Disagree**				**Agree**
	1	2	3	4	5
Describe the physician's role in home care and responsibilities in development and oversight of the home care plan.	**Disagree**				**Agree**
	1	2	3	4	5
Determine the appropriateness of a patient for home care.	**Disagree**				**Agree**
	1	2	3	4	5
Determine how, when and what services need to be implemented to provide quality care for the patient at home (home health services, homemaker, private duty, DME, palliative care and hospice, VA services, telehealth, etc.)	**Disagree**				**Agree**
	1	2	3	4	5
Explain how quality care transitions and coordinated health care services can reduce hospital admissions.	**Disagree**				**Agree**
	1	2	3	4	5
Describe medical ethics and legal and regulatory issues pertaining to the home care patient.	**Disagree**				**Agree**
	1	2	3	4	5

As a result of participating in this educational activity:

☐   I will change my practice.   How?

☐   I will not change my practice.   Why?   ☐ This activity reinforced my current practice.
         ☐ Other (please explain):

☐   I do not have a clinical practice.

I perceived commercial bias in this activity.   ☐ **Yes**   ☐ **No**
("Commercial bias" is defined as a personal judgment in favor of a specific proprietary business interest of an entity that produces, markets, sells or distributes healthcare goods or services consumed by, or used on, patients.)

If "yes," please comment:

Overall, I would rate this activity:	**Poor**				**Excellent**
	1	2	3	4	5

Other comments, suggestions or recommendations for future activities:

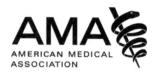

AMA
AMERICAN MEDICAL
ASSOCIATION

CME ACTIVITY PARTICIPATION RECORD
Medical Management of the Home Care Patient, 4ᵗʰ Edition

Only **physician participants** (MD, DO, or equivalent international medical degree) are eligible to receive *AMA PRA Category 1 Credit*™. Physicians will receive a certificate of credit, indicating one credit for each hour of participation, rounded to the nearest quarter credit (or hour). **Certificates will be emailed to participants who claim credit.** Physicians must complete this form to receive *AMA PRA Category 1 Credit*™. **Non-physician participants** may complete this form to obtain a certificate of participation indicating that this activity was approved for *AMA PRA Category 1 Credit*™.

Check one: ☐ *Physician*   ☐ *Non-Physician: Please email me a certificate of participation.*

Last name																						

First Name																						

Degree(s)																						

Organization																						

Street Address																						

City						State		Zip				

Telephone							Fax					

Email Address *(required for certificate delivery)*	@																					

FOR PHYSICIANS ONLY:

TOTAL CREDITS CLAIMED (not to exceed 3.5 credits): _____

☐ U.S. Licensed Physician   Medical Education Number*: _____

☐ Non-U.S. Licensed Physician   Year of birth**: _____

Specialty: _____

The medical education [ME] number is an 11-digit number assigned to every physician in the US by the AMA for identification and recording of basic information. The ME number is found on the AMA membership card.

** *Year of birth assists in uniquely identifying physicians for purposes of credit processing*

Signature   *Date*